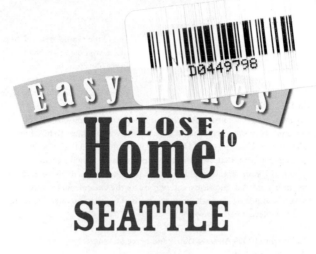

Easy Hikes
CLOSE to
Home
SEATTLE

including
Bellevue and Outlying Areas

ANDREW WEBER
AND
BRYCE STEVENS

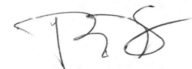

MENASHA RIDGE PRESS
Birmingham, Alabama

This book is meant only as a guide to select trails in the Seattle area and does not guarantee hiker safety in any way—you hike at your own risk. Neither Menasha Ridge Press nor Andrew Weber or Bryce Stevens is liable for property loss or damage, personal injury, or death that result in any way from accessing or hiking the trails described in the following pages. Please be aware that hikers have been injured in the Seattle area. Be especially cautious when walking on or near boulders, steep inclines, and drop-offs, and do not attempt to explore terrain that may be beyond your abilities. To help ensure an uneventful hike, please read carefully the introduction to this book, and perhaps get further safety information and guidance from other sources. Familiarize yourself thoroughly with the areas you intend to visit before venturing out. Ask questions, and prepare for the unforeseen. Familiarize yourself with current weather reports, maps of the area you intend to visit, and any relevant park regulations.

Copyright © 2009 Andrew Weber and Bryce Stevens
All rights reserved
Printed in the United States of America
Published by Menasha Ridge Press
Distributed by Publishers Group West
First edition, first printing

ISBN 978-0-89732-697-1

Cover by Scott McGrew
Cover photo by Andrew Weber
Text design by Annie Long
Maps by Andrew Weber, Bryce Stevens, and Steve Jones
All interior photos by Andrew Weber and Bryce Stevens

Menasha Ridge Press
P.O. Box 43673
Birmingham, AL 35243
www.menasharidge.com

Contents

4   **ABOUT THE AUTHORS**

5   **INTRODUCTION**

7   **TRAIL RECOMMENDATIONS**

9   **SEATTLE PARKS**

10   **Hike 1**: Camp Long
15   **Hike 2**: Carkeek Park
21   **Hike 3**: Discovery Park: Beaches, Bluffs, and Lighthouse
26   **Hike 4**: Schmitz Preserve Park
30   **Hike 5**: Seward Park
35   **Hike 6**: Washington Park Arboretum and Foster Island Trail

40   **BELLEVUE AND THE EAST SIDE**

41   **Hike 7**: Mercer Slough and Bellefields Nature Parks
46   **Hike 8**: Saint Edward State Park
50   **Hike 9**: O. O. Denny County Park Loop
54   **Hike 10**: Redmond Watershed Park and Preserve
58   **Hike 11**: Coal Creek Park
63   **Hike 12**: Cougar Mountain Regional Wildland Park:
       Wilderness Creek and Wilderness Peak Loop

67   **OUTLYING AREAS**

68   **Hike 13**: Rattlesnake Ledge
72   **Hike 14**: Little Si Trail
76   **Hike 15**: Twin Falls Natural Area and Olallie State Park
81   **Hike 16**: Spencer Island Natural Wildlife Reserve
86   **Hike 17**: Meadowdale County Park and Beach
90   **Hike 18**: Point Defiance Park

About the Authors

Andrew Weber

Thanks to a family scattered around the globe, Andrew Weber has become a world traveler for life, counting the Canadian Rockies, the beaches of New Zealand, and the deserts of southern Africa among his favorite places. He has been exploring the outdoors of the Pacific Northwest for more than a decade, including a successful climb of Mount Rainier in 2005 and a solo circumnavigation of the Wonderland Trail around the mountain in 2002. He currently resides in Seattle, where he works as a Web publisher and a freelance journalist and photographer. Andrew has written about a wide range of topics, including cultural events, the arts, the National Basketball Association and the National Football League.

Bryce Stevens

A lifelong Washingtonian, Bryce Stevens grew up in the Yakima area, graduated from the University of Washington, and has lived in Seattle for two decades. He has thoroughly explored the Cascade Range, the Olympic Mountains, and the lowlands of Puget Sound, all while hiking, backpacking, climbing, mountain biking, backcountry snowboarding, and sea kayaking. He discovered his love of outdoor photography while canyoneering in southeastern Utah in 2001 and has returned to the spectacular region every year since. In 1999 he cofounded **www.trails.com,** an online trail-information resource and topographic-mapping service that he continues to help run today. Bryce lives in the Maple Leaf neighborhood of Seattle with his wife, Julie, and their two sons, Kyle and Andrew.

Introduction

Welcome to *Easy Hikes Close to Home: Seattle*. This title in the *Easy Hikes* series is organized according to three Greater Seattle regions: Seattle Parks; Bellevue and the East Side; and Outlying Areas.

Numbered map icons on the inside front cover locate each primary trailhead and are keyed to the table of contents and narrative text for each trail. On the inside back cover, a map legend defines symbols for parking, restrooms, trail features, and other details. Armed with this handy guidebook, you can quickly head out the door and, well, take a hike!

Overview

Mileage shown for each hike corresponds to the total distance from start to finish, for loops, out-and-backs, figure eights, or a combination of shapes. You can shorten or extend some of them with connecting trails.

Trail Maps

Maps for each hike include GPS coordinates. Based on data downloaded from the author's handheld GPS unit and and plotted onto a digital U.S. Geological Survey (USGS) topo map, the coordinates are shown in two formats—as latitude/longitude and as UTM (Universal Transverse Mercator) coordinates.

HIKING ESSENTIALS

Boots should be your footwear of choice. Sport sandals are popular, but they leave much of your foot exposed and vulnerable to hazardous plants, thorns, rocks, and sharp twigs.

When it comes to water, err on the side of excess. Hydrate prior to your hike, carry (and drink) six ounces of water for every mile you plan to hike, and hydrate after the hike. Pack along a couple of small bottles even for short hikes. You may decide to linger on the trail, or take an alternate route and extend your time outdoors.

Always plan for unpredictable scenarios by carrying these items, in addition to water:

Map	Flashlight with extra batteries
Compass	Rain protection and a sweater or windbreaker, even in warm weather
Basic first-aid supplies, such as Band-Aids and aspirin	
Knife	Sun protection
Windproof matches or a lighter and fire starter	Insect repellent
	Whistle
Snacks	

GENERAL TIPS

The whole point of your outing is to enjoy nature, fresh air, and exercise. Here are a few tips to enhance your excursion:

- Avoid weekends and traditional holidays if possible; otherwise, go early in the morning. Trails that are packed in the summer are often clear during the colder months and during rainy times (but never hike during a thunderstorm).

- Before you hit the trail, double-check your map, and don't set out on the trail until you have the information you need.

- Once on the trail, be careful at overlooks, stay back from the edge of outcrops, and be absolutely sure of your footing wherever you are.

- Hike on open trails only. Respect trail and road closures, avoid trespassing on private land, and obtain permits if required. Leave gates as you found them or as marked.

- Stay on the existing trail, and avoid any littering.

- When hiking with children, use common sense to judge a child's capacity to hike a particular trail, and expect that the child may tire and need to be carried. Make sure children are adequately clothed for the weather, have proper shoes, and are protected from the sun with sunscreen. Kids dehydrate quickly, so make sure you have plenty of fluids for everyone.

- Take your time along the trails, whether you are doing one of this guide's short hikes or hours-long treks. In other words: Don't miss the trees for the forest. You may finish some of the "hike times" long before or after that suggested in the Overview box. A short-distance hike with a lot of up-and-downs may take more time and energy than a longer, flatter hike.

- Participate in some online wildlife observation counts. Cornell Lab of Ornithology operates **www.ebird.org** where you can login for free and submit bird lists or find out what's being seen at some of the area's birding hot spots. A similar count is being done for butterflies at **www.wisconsinbutterflies.org/butterflies/sightings.**

- Never spook animals. An unannounced approach, a sudden movement, or a loud noise startles most animals, and a surprised animal can be dangerous. Give them plenty of space.

- Be courteous to others you encounter on the trails.

- Look up! Keep an eye out for standing dead trees and storm-damaged living trees with loose or broken limbs that can fall at any time.

- Know your ability, and carry necessary supplies for changes in weather or other conditions.

TRAIL RECOMMENDATIONS

Hikes with Mountain-Biking Opportunities

08 Saint Edward State Park
10 Redmond Watershed Park and Preserve
17 Meadowdale County Park and Beach

Hikes with Waterfalls

11 Coal Creek Park
15 Twin Falls Natural Area and Olallie State Park

Hikes on Lakes

05 Seward Park
06 Washington Park Arboretum and Foster Island Trail
08 Saint Edward State Park
13 Rattlesnake Ledge

Hikes along Rivers and Streams

07 Mercer Slough and Bellefields Nature Parks
15 Twin Falls Natural Area and Olallie State Park
16 Spencer Island Natural Wildlife Reserve

Hikes with Historic Sites

01 Camp Long
03 Discovery Park: Beaches, Bluffs, and Lighthouse
11 Coal Creek Park
18 Point Defiance Park

Scenic Hikes

All hikes in this guide were chosen for their scenic qualities.

Hikes with Bird-Watching

06 Washington Park Arboretum and Foster Island Trail
07 Mercer Slough and Bellefields Nature Parks
16 Spencer Island Natural Wildlife Reserve

Good Hikes for Runners

03 Discovery Park: Beaches, Bluffs, and Lighthouse
05 Seward Park
08 Saint Edward State Park
10 Redmond Watershed Park and Preserve
11 Coal Creek Park
12 Cougar Mountain Regional Wildland Park
15 Twin Falls Natural Area and Olallie State Park
18 Point Defiance Park

Hikes with Old-Growth Forest

04 Schmitz Preserve Park
05 Seward Park
09 O. O. Denny County Park Loop
18 Point Defiance Park

Hikes with Great Viewpoints

13 Rattlesnake Ledge
14 Little Si Trail
18 Point Defiance Park

Year-round Hikes

All hikes in this guide are great year-round.

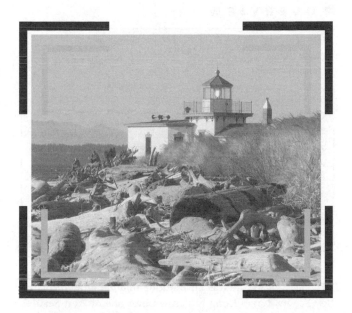

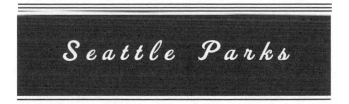

Seattle Parks

■ OVERVIEW

LENGTH: 1.1 miles	**MAPS:** USGS Seattle South
CONFIGURATION: Loop with many side-trip options available	**FACILITIES:** Restrooms and water at visitor center
SCENERY: Picturesque pond, stream, and fields; seasonal views of Seattle	**SPECIAL COMMENTS:** Historic Boy Scout camp with old lodge and cabins for rent; climbing rock; and glacier-roping practice course. To rent one of the cabins or shelters, the Environmental Learning Center, or the fire circle, contact the Camp Long office via the Internet at www.seattle.gov/parks/environment/camplong.htm or call (206) 684-7434. Information on open hours, equipment rentals, and climbing classes on Schurman Rock is also available.
EXPOSURE: Mostly shaded	
TRAFFIC: Moderate	
TRAIL SURFACE: Dirt, gravel, and paved	
HIKING TIME: 1–2 hours	
ACCESS: Hikable year-round, Tuesday–Sunday, 10 a.m.–6 p.m.; closed on Sundays December–February; no fee for parking or park access	

■ SNAPSHOT

Originally established as an outdoor training ground for the Boy Scouts, Camp Long has grown into one of West Seattle's premier parks. The scouting facilities were opened to the general public in 1984. Ever since then, everyone has been welcome to hike the trails, camp in the shelters, and even climb on famous Schurman Rock, where many serious Cascade mountaineers first tested and developed their skills.

■ CLOSE-UP

At just less than 70 acres, Camp Long is far from a significant park if measured by size alone. Yet, as the old saying goes, good things come in small packages. For density of attractions, few parks can match this often-overlooked West Seattle reserve.

All outings at Camp Long should start at the visitor center. Built by the Works Progress Administration (WPA) during

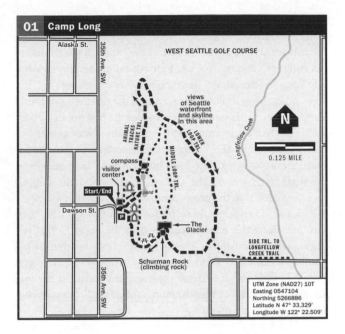

01 Camp Long

Alaska St.

35th Ave. SW

WEST SEATTLE GOLF COURSE

views
of Seattle
waterfront
and skyline
in this area

ANIMAL TRACKS NATURE TRL.

LOWER LOOP TRL.

MIDDLE LOOP TRL.

Longfellow Creek

N

0.125 MILE

compass
visitor
center

Start/End

pond

Dawson St.

P

The
Glacier

SIDE TRL. TO
LONGFELLOW
CREEK TRAIL

Schurman Rock
(climbing rock)

35th Ave. SW

UTM Zone (NAD27) 10T
Easting 0547104
Northing 5266886
Latitude N 47° 33.329'
Longitude W 122° 22.509'

the Great Depression, the structure was modeled after Oregon's
Multnomah Falls Lodge, which was completed more than a
decade earlier in 1925; the heavy stones used in construction at
Camp Long had once paved Seattle's E Madison Street, which
was being resurfaced at the time.

Growing right next to the lodge door is an interpretive
garden of native plants, modeling a forest-edge plant community typical of the area. Ecologists call this type of environment
an ecotone, the meeting of two different landscapes to create a
particularly high diversity of species. (The same phenomenon
occurs in oceans, when unusual densities of marine life congre-
gate where warm and cold currents mix together.) Many of the
plants visible in Camp Long's ecotone can also be seen in the
interior of the park.

Inside the visitor center, you'll find information on the history and natural environment of the park on a series of helpful displays. The facility also features a great hall (to the left of the entrance) that is often used for educational gatherings and also hosts the occasional wedding or other ceremony.

An easily completed loop around the perimeter of Camp Long on a series of named trails provides the best hiking option. To get started, circle around the back of the visitor center and pass by several of the camping cabins. Much like the lodge itself, these buildings built by the WPA, using reclaimed materials from around the city as part of an environmental recycling ethic that the camp continues to promote today.

Head down a gentle slope toward Polliwog Pond, then turn left along the service road next to the water to find the beginning of the Animal Tracks Nature Trail, in front of the number-seven cabin (also known as "St. Helens"). Here you should look for a giant stone compass sunk into the ground, another WPA project built to help young Boy Scouts develop wilderness-navigation skills.

The Animal Tracks Nature Trail, which follows a ridge to the northern end of the park, offers occasional views of downtown Seattle, the docks at Harbor Island, and the Space Needle through gaps in the trees. (The forest is a mix of red alder, big leaf maple, and various other species, including western red cedar, although there is no old growth; the understory is characterized by sword ferns, ivy, Oregon grape, and blackberry bushes.) The trail bends sharply around to the right at its northern point and heads downhill. Stay to the left at a junction with the Middle Loop Trail (the general rule for hiking the perimeter in the clockwise direction) and cross a tributary of Longfellow Creek, the outflow from the wetlands next to the pond you saw at the outset.

At a second junction stay left again to join the Lower Loop Trail, which runs along the eastern edge of the park closest to the West Seattle Golf Course. Red foxes, frequently spotted on the nearby golf-course grounds, can sometimes be observed here as well.

Shortly before the Lower Loop Trail ends, a narrow, unmarked trail heads into the trees to the left. This junction connects Camp Long to the Longfellow Creek Trail, a 4-mile-long urban creek corridor through West Seattle; it provides an option for anyone wishing to add to their total hiking distance, although the route frequently travels along roads and sidewalks.

Past the junction, the trail climbs up a short hill to reach the bottom of "The Glacier," a manufactured-rock surface where climbers are likely to be practicing their rope and ice-travel techniques. The Glacier is an add-on to Schurman Rock, just up the stone steps to the left, which tends to be the focus of more-advanced climbing and belaying activity.

Schurman Rock is named for Camp Long cofounder and scout leader Clark Schurman, who envisioned creating a climbing surface that emulated many different types of rocks and challenges typical of the Olympic and Cascade ranges, and for whom Camp Schurman on Mount Rainier's Emmons Glacier is also named. Completed in 1939, Schurman was the first artificial climbing rock in North America. And it has been the staging ground for many great young climbers who later moved on to bigger things. The rock got a major face-lift in 2003, thanks to a consortium of public and private outdoor groups, so it will continue to help train climbers long into the future. In fact, some of them may be practicing on the day of your hike, making the picnic tables and grassy area next to the rock a great place to relax and watch them at work. When you are ready to wrap up your hike, cross the lawn to reach the service road through the trees, and follow it back to the parking lot.

■ MORE FUN

The West Seattle Golf Course, adjacent to Camp Long to the east, once hosted the 1953 U.S. Amateur Public Links Championships and has a beautiful layout with great views of downtown Seattle. To schedule a tee time or get more information, visit the West Seattle Golf Club on the Web at **seattle golf.com/west-seattle.php** or by phone at (206) 935-5187.

■ TO THE TRAILHEAD

From Interstate 5 just south of downtown Seattle, take Exit 163A, West Seattle Bridge—Columbian Way. Stay to the right on the off-ramp and continue onto the West Seattle Bridge, which becomes Fauntleroy Way SW when it ascends up to West Seattle. At the first traffic light, turn left onto 35th Avenue SW and drive about 0.5 miles up the hill to SW Dawson Street. At this intersection, turn left into Camp Long and continue through the gate to the parking lot on the right.

■ OVERVIEW

LENGTH: 3.5 miles around perimeter	**HIKING TIME:** 1–2 hours or longer with side trips
CONFIGURATION: Figure 8 with several options	**ACCESS:** Hikable year-round, daily, 6 a.m.–10 p.m.; no fees for parking or park access
SCENERY: Wildlife, woodlands, beach, and sea life	
EXPOSURE: Wooded park with many shady areas	**MAPS:** Printed maps on information board near bridge over the railroad tracks, USGS Seattle North
TRAFFIC: Busy often, but South Ridge trails see little traffic	**FACILITIES:** Restrooms and water near the northern park play area
TRAIL SURFACE: Mixture of gravel, dirt, boardwalk, and paved	

■ SNAPSHOT

Occupying a stretch of Puget Sound shoreline in northwestern Seattle, Carkeek Park presents a mix of well-developed fields and play areas, an extensive network of trails, and a wide expanse of rocky beach to explore. High bluffs above the water allow all comers to enjoy views usually reserved for the residents of the upscale Blue Ridge neighborhood where the park is nestled.

■ CLOSE-UP

Carkeek is no secret to many Seattle residents. On any weekend in good weather, expect to compete for space on the playing fields and for parking. People come here for good reason: The park has a variety of attractions, and despite the crowds plenty of peace and solitude can be found out on the trails by anyone willing to put forth a little effort.

From the entrance, the road winds through woods and fields to the upper parking lot next to the playground. If this lot is full, various other less-formal parking opportunities can be

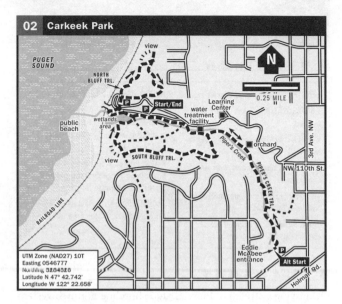

02   Carkeek Park

view

PUGET
SOUND

NORTH
BLUFF TRL.

N

0.25 MILE

Learning
Center

water
treatment
facility

Start/End

public
beach

wetlands
area

Piper's Creek

orchard

3rd Ave. NW

view

SOUTH BLUFF TRL.

PIPER'S CREEK TRL.

NW 110th St.

RAILROAD LINE

Eddie
McAbee
entrance

Alt Start

Holman Rd.

UTM Zone (NAD27) 10T
Easting 0546777
Northing 5284510
Latitude N 47° 42.742'
Longitude W 122° 22.658'

found farther along the one-way loop road. There is sure to be space somewhere.

Many visitors never venture too far beyond their cars. Adjacent to the parking lot are grass fields that host frequent volleyball, softball, and Frisbee games, and a group of public picnic areas with outdoor grills also stands nearby. A charming playground, which features a slide where kids pass through a giant salmon, will keep children occupied for hours.

Several hiking opportunities are available from the upper parking lot. Despite Carkeek's limited size, the woods north and south of the park road are interlaced with a substantial network of trails. It is possible to get disoriented with so many options, but because of the restricted space no one will stay lost for very long. The easiest way to see the park is to explore on your own; a pamphlet with a trail map should be available at a billboard in the southwest corner of the upper parking lot, next to the beach-access bridge.

Note that Seattle Parks and Recreation is trying to decrease the number of informal trails by specifically graveling maintained trails and letting the rest return to nature, so try to stay on the official trails if you can. Bicycles are allowed only on the Piper's Creek Trail. And dogs are forbidden on the beach and must be leashed at all times everywhere else.

The Beach

From the upper playfield, you can access Carkeek Park's beach via a footbridge that crosses some railroad tracks. Kids are sure to be delighted if a train thunders underneath, especially because the vantage offers the chance to see the speeding cars up close, an impressive sight since many freight trains stretch more than a mile in length.

The view west from the beach encompasses Bainbridge Island and the Kitsap Peninsula with the jagged Olympic Mountains beyond. All kinds of boats—from small day-sailers to giant tankers making for the Strait of Juan de Fuca—provide perspective.

The beach sits on Puget Sound, and the water is too cold for an extended swim (though a quick dip or wade can provide relief on a hot summer day). Exploration, therefore, is the main attraction for many park users. Low tide reveals crabs, anemones, starfish, and many other small marine animals hidden in the tide pools and among the rocks. And the exposed sand allows you to wander up or down the shoreline, possibly as far as Golden Gardens Park over a mile away on Shilshole Bay to the southwest.

The North Bluff

To reach the northern side of the park, look for a trailhead along the fence behind the picnic tables. The gravel trail climbs quickly onto the North Bluff, where several viewpoints open above the cliff and expose the steep drop to the beach below. The trail eventually dead-ends at the North Meadow, an open grassy area on a hill with a remarkable view of the sound. Houses are visible nearby, too, as the meadow borders on private property.

Retreat a short distance and you'll find wooden stairs down to the left. Descend into darker woods, composed largely of big leaf maples and red alders; ferns, salal, and other undergrowth cover the forest floor along the route.

Complete the obvious perimeter loop (no more than 0.7 miles) to return to the park road and then to your car. Various spur trails lead through the center of the loop and can be used to lengthen your hike.

Piper's Creek and the South Ridge

The most extensive hiking opportunities at Carkeek are found on the Piper's Creek Trail and the adjoining trails of the South Ridge. Piper's Creek flows through the center of the park, emptying into Puget Sound, and its namesake trail runs alongside for about 1 mile up to an alternate park entrance.

The trail starts just below the upper parking lot; look for a footpath sign and some steps downward. As with the North Bluff, there are many options here. You will know when you have reached Piper's Creek, though, and the right trail is easy to find.

A small wetland lies at the mouth of the creek. The trail surface turns to boardwalk to pass through the lowland bog, with its carpet of algae and high reeds, before returning to gravel. Chum and coho salmon run the creek to spawn in season, an amazing spectacle given the creek's minimal flow and the heavy development nearby.

After following the edge of the grassy lower meadow for about 0.3 miles, the trail passes a small water-treatment plant, then enters a broad ravine. The second-growth forest here is similar in composition to the woods on the North Bluff, although the occasional giant stump testifies to the size of the western red cedars and western hemlocks that grew here before being cut down in the early 20th century.

Upon entering the ravine, the trail starts a gradual uphill climb. Soon some apple trees appear on the left, marking the remnants of the Piper Homestead Orchard. A. W. Piper, the land's owner, was a politician and artist who opened a bakery and candy company in 1876. He and his wife, Minna, sold produce and flowers they grew in the orchard from a wagon in Pike Place Market downtown until the property was sold and developed into a park in 1929.

The trail continues its steady ascent for another half mile until reaching the head of the ravine at the Eddie McAbee Park entrance on NW 100th Place. There is only room for a few cars here, but this side entry can be a great alternate access to the park.

Return down Piper's Creek Trail to just before the water-treatment facility and find the South Ridge Trail to the left. Even on a busy summer day you can expect to have this area of the park to yourself. This trail leads uphill to the southern edge of the ravine, then winds along the top of the ridge back toward the beach. Many side paths lead off into the adjacent residential area as the trail negotiates a series of short rises. Other spurs lead back down to Piper's Creek, but it is easy to stay on the ridge.

After a half mile you will reach the South Bluff and a high overlook. There is no doubt you are at the park boundary, as you emerge from the trees and find yourself practically in someone's backyard. Find the South Bluff Trail, which drops quickly through the woods along the top of the cliff. Be careful here, especially if you have children with you—the sharp drop-off to the beach and sandy tread can be hazardous. From the bottom of the South Bluff it is an easy walk back to your car.

■ MORE FUN

Visit the Carkeek Park Environmental Learning Center at 950 NW Carkeek Park Road, near the park's main entrance. The building offers a host of environmental education and stewardship activities, and as the first building in the City of Seattle rated "Gold-Level" in the U.S. Green Building Council's Leadership in Energy and Environmental Design (LEED) system, it practices what it preaches. Check the Web site for hours and more information: **www.seattle.gov/parks/parkspaces/ CarkeekPark/ELC.htm.**

■ TO THE TRAILHEAD

Starting on I-5 north of downtown Seattle, take Exit 173. At the end of the ramp, turn left onto 1 Ave NE and then turn left again at the next light onto Northgate Way, headed west. Northgate Way eventually becomes N 105th Street and continues across WA 99. At the next major intersection after WA 99, cross Greenwood Avenue and veer slightly left onto Holman Road. In a short distance at a sign for Carkeek Park, turn right onto Third Avenue NW. Then turn left onto NW 110th Street, which soon becomes NW Carkeek Park Road. From here, signs guide you into the parking areas of Carkeek Park and the one-way loop road. Park in the upper lot nearest the beach or continue down to the lower parking lot.

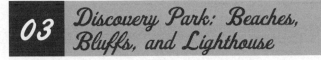

03 *Discovery Park: Beaches, Bluffs, and Lighthouse*

■ OVERVIEW

LENGTH: 3 miles (round-trip)	**TRAFFIC:** High
CONFIGURATION: Loop with many options to extend the hike	**TRAIL SURFACE:** Mixture of dirt, pavement, gravel, and boardwalk
SCENERY: Historic Fort Lawton grounds, sandy beaches, lighthouse; views of Puget Sound, Seattle, and Mount Rainier	**HIKING TIME:** 2–4 hours
	ACCESS: Hikable year-round; no fees for parking or park access
EXPOSURE: Shaded on upper trails; exposed on beach trails	**MAPS:** USGS Seattle North
	FACILITIES: Restrooms and water at trailhead

■ SNAPSHOT

Occupying a prominent point between Shilshole and Elliott bays, this former military installation is the largest park in the city of Seattle. Blessed with 534 acres of forests, fields, bluffs, and beaches, and even a picturesque lighthouse with excellent views of northern Puget Sound, Discovery Park is a great destination for the entire family.

■ CLOSE-UP

Discovery Park has more than 10 miles of trails, including a prominently marked Loop Trail that circles most of the open fields and old military housing in the park's southern end. However, because this trail never reaches the beach—arguably the park's leading attraction—a better and more representative loop is described here. This hike descends through the wooded areas in the northern half of the park, travels along the beach to the lighthouse, then returns up the bluff, offering many options for further exploration along the way.

From the North Parking Lot, begin by heading west along the paved road, which is closed to vehicles. Stay on this road

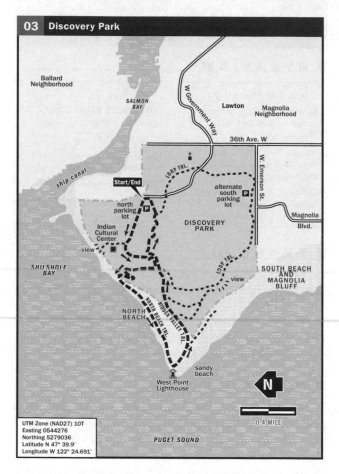

03   Discovery Park

Ballard
Neighborhood

SALMON
BAY

W Government Way

Lawton

Magnolia
Neighborhood

36th Ave. W

ship canal

LOOP TRL

Start/End

north
parking
lot

W. Emerson St.

alternate
south
parking
lot

DISCOVERY
PARK

Indian
Cultural
Center

view

Magnolia
Blvd.

SHILSHOLE
BAY

LOOP TRL

view

SOUTH BEACH
AND
MAGNOLIA
BLUFF

HIDDEN VALLEY TRL.

NORTH
BEACH

NORTH BEACH TRL.

sandy
beach

N

West Point
Lighthouse

0.4 MILE

UTM Zone (NAD27) 10T
Easting 0544276
Northing 5279036
Latitude N 47° 39.9'
Longitude W 122° 24.691'

PUGET SOUND

through the first junction at the end of the grassy picnic area,
where another road branches to the left.

A second junction in the road heads up a small rise to the
Daybreak Star Indian Cultural Center. Run by the United Indi-
ans of All Tribes Foundation (UIATF), this organization provides social services to Native Americans. The site for the

Cultural Center was obtained following a heated standoff between Native American activists and the U.S. government in the spring of 1970 after the military decommissioned Fort Lawton. Bernie Whitebear, a former Green Beret and longtime advocate for Native American causes, led a so-called invasion and occupation of the fort, arguing that the property was on historic Native American land. The city of Seattle, however, wanted to turn Fort Lawton into a public park. After several months and significant media attention, a compromise agreement was reached, ceding 20 acres of the newly formed Discovery Park to the UIATF with a 99-year renewable lease from the city. Whitebear went on to head the UIATF for three decades, until his death in 2000 at the age of 62.

The Cultural Center's striking architecture blends modern and traditional Native American design, and offers an impressive view from a high bluff out over Shilshole Bay, making it a quick and worthy side trip. Simply follow the road around to the northern side of the building—its best façade—and look for a wooden overlook platform on the far side of the lawn. From this viewpoint, the masts at Shilshole Marina resemble a forest of thin trees near the Lake Washington Ship Canal entrance; on a clear day Mount Baker can be seen far away to the north.

After this short detour, continue back on the main road, which curves around to the left and starts heading south. About a quarter mile past the Cultural Center, the official Loop Trail intersects the road. Turn right on the Loop Trail until you reach a second road, then turn right again and follow the road back to the north, close to where it dead-ends. This somewhat awkward, roundabout route is the result of a landslide that washed away a better access path sometime in the past.

On the opposite side of a small picnic area to the left is a gap in a chain-link fence with a green wooden post and a sign directing hikers to the North Beach Trail. Follow this path as it descends through trees on a steep trail with some wooden stairs, bending to the right and dropping 200 feet in about an eighth of a mile.

The trail turns left, above a long breakwater of heavy boulders, along the shore toward the lighthouse. Even with only moderate wind, sizable swells often crash against the rocks here, despite the short run of open water and considerable shelter provided by Bainbridge Island and the Kitsap Peninsula across Puget Sound.

After a half mile, the breakwater gives way to a stretch of sandy beach below the lighthouse. The trail cuts inland, but the beach itself provides a more interesting way to get around the point, except during bad weather or at extreme high tide. Lots of shells, driftwood, and other flotsam lie on the sand, providing fun for beachcombers of all ages who search for treasures along the shore. Marine wildlife—including crabs, barnacles, starfish, and sea anemones—is frequently visible at low tide. This approach also provides excellent views of the lighthouse itself, known as the West Point Lighthouse, and its attached radar installation.

The far side of the point (where the sandy beach continues southeast for another half mile) has treasures all its own, offering interesting views of West Seattle, Mount Rainier, Puget Sound, and the Olympic Mountains. This area is known as the South Beach, and it is certainly worth exploring. Be wary of the tides, though, as people have been known to get trapped here below the steep walls of Magnolia Bluff.

When you are ready to continue hiking, look for the trail heading uphill on the northern side of the lighthouse access road. The path follows the road for a few hundred yards before reaching a junction (signed for the Hidden Valley Trail) across from an excellent viewpoint over South Beach from the top of the bluff.

Take the Hidden Valley Trail and climb up through the woods, crossing several intersections until it ends on the park's official Loop Trail, just short of another road. Note that once you cross this road, you are back on the same short section of the Loop Trail you hiked earlier, except now you're traveling in the opposite direction.

Stay on the Loop Trail as it winds up and down through a pleasant forest for a half mile and crosses two more paved roads (long closed to traffic) in one of the nicest sections of the upper park. At a third paved road, head left down the hill to return to the North Parking Lot, where you began.

To extend your hike, the best bet is to follow the official Loop Trail as far as you wish to go, potentially adding several more miles if you complete the entire circuit. Another option is to take the South Beach Trail away from the beach rather than the Hidden Valley Trail, as described earlier, then continue all the way around the Loop Trail in a counterclockwise direction. This will allow you to see the open southern half of the park without ever having to retrace your steps.

■ TO THE TRAILHEAD

From I-5 north of downtown Seattle, take Exit 169, NE 45th Street, and drive west. Continuing west, 45th Street becomes 46th Street, then drops down into the city of Ballard and becomes Market Street. In Ballard, go left on 15th Avenue NW and immediately cross the Ballard Bridge. Make the first right after the bridge onto W Emerson Street, then make another right onto Gilman Avenue W. Gilman Avenue W eventually becomes W Government Way and goes into the Discovery Park east entrance. Once inside the park, stay to the right and drive to the North Parking Lot.

04 Schmitz Preserve Park

■ OVERVIEW

LENGTH: 1 mile (round-trip; side trip options)	**TRAIL SURFACE:** Dirt, gravel, and some boardwalk
CONFIGURATION: Loop	**HIKING TIME:** 1–2 hours
SCENERY: Old-growth forest contrasted with enormous logging stumps in an urban park; a cascading stream	**ACCESS:** Hikable year-round; no fees for parking or park access
	MAPS: USGS Seattle South
EXPOSURE: Shaded	**FACILITIES:** No restroom or water facilities
TRAFFIC: Moderate	

■ SNAPSHOT

This unassuming little park hides a singular example of old-growth forest in the middle of the city. With a good network of trails through a quiet, secluded valley, Schmitz Preserve Park makes a great place for a quick escape to the woods, despite its limited size.

■ CLOSE-UP

A full century after it was established in 1908, Schmitz Park, originally a 30-acre parcel of land donated by Ferdinand and Emma Schmitz, remains true to its founders' intent—to be kept as an example of the local forest as it was discovered by Seattle's first settlers.

The pioneers of the Denny Party, who landed just down the hill at Alki Point in November 1851, would undoubtedly still feel at home in Schmitz, even if they would find the rest of Seattle completely unrecognizable. Ironically, the park has come to represent Seattle's past, though the name *Alki* comes from a Chinook word indicating the future.

Now expanded to more than 50 acres, Schmitz Park continues to protect the region's natural heritage. In fact, it does such

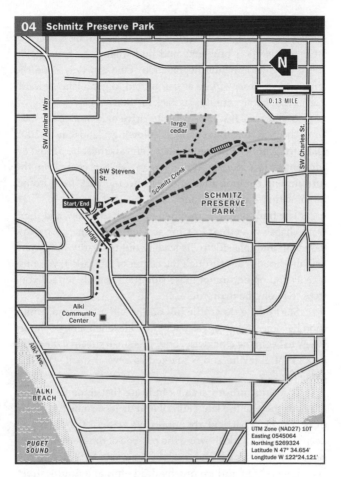

04 Schmitz Preserve Park

large cedar

SW Admiral Way

SW Charles St.

0.13 MILE

SW Stevens St.

Schmitz Creek

SCHMITZ PRESERVE PARK

Start/End P

bridge

Alki Community Center

Alki Ave.

ALKI BEACH

PUGET SOUND

UTM Zone (NAD27) 10T
Easting 0545064
Northing 5269324
Latitude N 47° 34.654'
Longitude W 122°24.121'

a good job that the University of Washington Forestry Department uses the park as a prime example of Pacific Northwest old-growth forest, proudly displaying it to visiting Asian forest managers. The future of the global environment will undoubtedly be determined in Asia, home to more than half of the world's population and most of its fastest growing economies. Already today, dust clouds from desertification in western China occasionally reach the U.S. Pacific Coast, exacerbating smog and other air-pollution problems and underlining the truly global effects of environmental degradation. One can only hope the university's visitors will be as committed to good land stewardship as the Schmitz family was back in 1908.

At one time it was possible to drive on a road to the center of the park, but that changed following a landslide in 2002 that gave Schmitz a makeover. Now all cars must be parked on adjacent surface streets, although many visitors come from the surrounding communities and walk to the park from home, forgoing their cars altogether.

The trails here are unsigned but easy to follow, and there is no chance of getting lost for any length of time. A narrow loop with multiple side trails leading out to nearby streets and neighborhoods runs through the center of the park. If you mistakenly end up on one of these side trails, simply retrace your steps to rejoin the main route.

Start hiking down the hill on the old gravel road, which soon becomes a dirt single-track trail. Head left along Schmitz Creek to begin the clockwise loop; this small stream defines the park's central ravine and is marked by several small waterfalls along the way.

A few mammoth stumps indicate that minimal logging did occur here in the late 1800s. Nonetheless, some truly giant trees remain. A particularly impressive western red cedar—its deeply grooved bark showing the passage of time—stands on a rise on a spur trail, which leaves the main trail to the left from a large intersection and eventually dead-ends at a nearby street. Watch for other ancient trees with blackened bark, revealing forest fires that swept through West Seattle in years past.

A boardwalk runs through the wetlands along the creek, winding through skunk cabbage, water parsley, and various ferns. Metal laths on the elevated boards help keep the footing secure even when the surface is wet, which is most of the time because of the shelter and cooling shade of the tree canopy.

The trail reaches the southern end of the park then doubles back to the right, climbing the valley wall. Pileated woodpeckers are common here, and can easily be heard or seen taking their toll on the trees nearby. The woodpeckers are only one of a large range of bird species that live in the mixed-conifer forest, which also is home to Steller's jays, song sparrows, and black-capped chickadees.

Eventually, the loop trail reaches an old road (now closed to vehicles) along the creek. Continue down the road to find a stairway on the left that'll take you to the Schmitz Park Bridge, built in 1936, overhead. Head up the stairs and cross the bridge to return to your car. The road continues under the bridge and heads downhill to the Alki Community Center, an alternate place to begin the hike.

■ TO THE TRAILHEAD

From I-5 just south of downtown Seattle, take Exit 163A, W Seattle Bridge—Columbian Way. Stay to the right on the off-ramp and continue onto the West Seattle Bridge. Take the Admiral Way exit, then continue for about 2 miles and turn left onto SW Stevens Street just before a bridge. Park along SW Stevens Street, and find the trailhead near the intersection with Admiral Way.

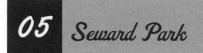

■ OVERVIEW

LENGTH: 4.6 miles (2.4 miles of paved shoreline trail and 2.2 miles of interior dirt trails)	**TRAIL SURFACE:** Dirt in interior, paved around perimeter
CONFIGURATION: Loop with options	**HIKING TIME:** 1–3 hours
SCENERY: Views of the surrounding area and Lake Washington; old-growth forest and other picturesque plant life; lakeshore beaches	**ACCESS:** Hikable year-round; no fees for parking or park access
	MAPS: USGS Seattle South and Bellevue South
EXPOSURE: Shaded on interior trails, exposed on shoreline trail	**FACILITIES:** Restrooms and water at the parking areas (some may be closed in winter)
TRAFFIC: Heavy on shoreline trail, moderate on interior trails	

■ SNAPSHOT

Before Lake Washington was lowered by the opening of the ship canal in 1917, the peninsula now occupied by Seward Park was almost an island. Today, the park is an island of a different sort. Resisting the Seattle development that has spread around it for almost a century, Seward is now one of the last significant vestiges of old-growth forest within the city limits. A paved circular loop follows the island's lakefront shoreline and connects to a network of single-track trails beneath the ancient trees.

■ CLOSE-UP

Seward Park was named for William Seward, who was appointed as secretary of state by Abraham Lincoln in 1861. An outspoken critic of slavery and an ardent supporter of the Union during the Civil War, Seward became a highly visible and symbolic enemy of the Confederacy. His further abuse of power as head of the government program to eliminate so-called disloyals in the North cemented his reputation among Southerners as a

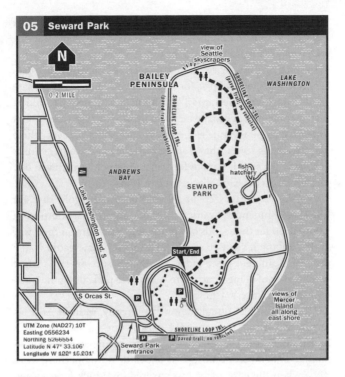

05   Seward Park

N

0.2 MILE

BAILEY
PENINSULA

view of
Seattle
skyscrapers

LAKE
WASHINGTON

SHORELINE LOOP TRL.
(paved trail; no vehicles)

SHORELINE LOOP TRL.
(paved trail; no vehicles)

ANDREWS
BAY

Lake Washington Blvd S

SEWARD
PARK

fish
hatchery

Start/End

S Orcas St.

P

P

views of
Mercer
Island
all along
east shore

UTM Zone (NAD27) 10T
Easting 0556234
Northing 5266554
Latitude N 47° 33.106'
Longitude W 122° 15.201'

SHORELINE LOOP TRL.

P (paved trail; no vehicles)

Seward Park
entrance

man to be feared and hated. In fact, Seward became a supple-
mental target of the assassination conspiracy organized by John
Wilkes Booth. On April 14, 1865, the same night Booth shot
Lincoln, a man named Lewis Powell stabbed Seward in the
throat in an attempt to kill him as well. Despite suffering very
serious wounds, Seward survived the attack and continued to
serve in his post as secretary of state under Andrew Johnson.
During Johnson's administration, Seward became well-known
for his pivotal role in the purchase of Alaska from Russia in the
spring of 1867. At the time, Alaska was generally considered a
frozen wasteland and the transaction was mocked as "Seward's
Folly," a monumental waste of taxpayer money.

Today, it's hard to see how the acquisition of Alaska for the paltry sum of $7.2 million could be viewed as anything but one of the greatest bargains in U.S. history. Seward obtained 360 million acres of land for two cents an acre, substantially less than Thomas Jefferson had paid for his celebrated Louisiana Purchase six decades before. Seward's $7.2 million outlay in 1867 would be the equivalent of approximately $90 million in 2009, an amount that Alaskan oil revenue alone repays approximately every three days. And this says nothing for the vast value of the other natural resources the state is famous for—including gold, which was first discovered in the Klondike in the late 1800s.

Most historians credit the ensuing Alaska gold rush for the establishment of Seattle as a major city, the last outpost of civilization for thousands of would-be prospectors on their way to the Yukon. It's safe to say that without Alaska, Seattle would be a very different place today. For that reason, Seward's name was worthy of being attached to a 300-acre park along the western shore of Lake Washington.

Ironically, although Seward indirectly spurred Seattle's urban expansion, his namesake park is one of the few places remaining in the city that development has never reached. It's hard to imagine from most parts of Seattle now, but there was a time when the entire area was covered in a thick forest—and Seward Park is one of the last remaining stands.

A 2.4-mile Shoreline Trail, following a paved road now closed to motor vehicles, loops around the perimeter of the park along the edge of Lake Washington. This route is very popular and provides views of the lake and the surrounding communities. Particularly interesting are some of the palatial houses visible on Mercer Island to the east; it wouldn't take many of these estates to top the $7.2 million price tag of Seward's entire Alaska purchase. Also, looking northward offers a view of some of the tallest skyscrapers downtown rising above the Mount Baker and Beacon Hill neighborhoods and the I-90 Bridge spanning the lake.

A fish hatchery on the eastern side of the park was constructed by the Works Progress Administration (WPA) during the New Deal to raise trout for stocking local lakes, including Lake Washington. The vision was for Seward Park to become a fisherman's paradise, but the reality has not quite lived up to those expectations. The fishery is not generally open to the public, although a new education center has been in the works for some time.

For most hikers, the primary attraction at Seward Park is its forest, which exhibits all of the required characteristics of old growth—standing snags, a layered canopy, fallen nurse logs, and some very large trees, among others. Although lacking any truly gigantic specimens, Seward Park harbors some trees that are up to 200 years old and contains one of the largest madrones in the state. Along with madrones, the lowland forest contains a mix of western red cedars, Douglas firs, western hemlocks, and big leaf maples. The maples are notable for their ability to host epiphytes (plants that grow on other plants) such as licorice ferns, mosses, and lichens. Unfortunately, English ivy, a foreign, invasive plant that chokes out endemic species, grows here as well. Volunteer groups are working in conjunction with park administration to eradicate the plant in an attempt to restore the natural ecosystem.

The best way to see the Seward Park is to find your own way around. The central spine of the park is laced with a series of dirt paths, seven separate segments (totaling 2.2 miles) linked on all sides to the Shoreline Trail. By following a mix of the interior trails and the Shoreline, this network can lead you to all corners of the park and its varied attractions. Thanks to the general topography and short distances involved, navigation is simple even for first time visitors. Note that dogs must be kept on leashes.

■ MORE FUN

Try the Columbia City Ale House for a posthike beer or meal. Part of the revitalization of the historic Columbia City community, this cozy neighborhood pub offers a wide variety of excellent local brews and often features special seasonal varieties. The Ale House, located at 4914 Rainier Avenue S, can be reached from Seward Park by following S Orcas Street until it intersects with Rainier Avenue and then turning right (north). For more information, call (206) 723-5123 or visit **www.seattlealehouses.com/ColumbiaCity/index.asp.**

■ TO THE TRAILHEAD

From I-5 in downtown Seattle, take Exit 164 onto I-90 East. Immediately exit onto Rainier Avenue S, Exit 3A, and turn right onto Rainier at the bottom of the ramp. Follow Rainier Avenue S about 3 miles through the historic downtown of Columbia City. After downtown, turn left (east) onto S Orcas Street, which eventually ends at Seward Park. Turn right into the park entrance, and park in one of the lower lots if you plan to walk the paved shoreline trail. Continue to the upper parking lot if you plan to hike the interior trails or if the lower lots are full.

Washington Park Arboretum and Foster Island Trail

■ OVERVIEW

LENGTH: 3.5 miles (1.5-mile loop in Arboretum; plus optional 2-mile round-trip out-and-back on Foster Island Trail)

CONFIGURATION: Loop with many options

SCENERY: Incredible display of plant life from around the world, island shoreline trails, territorial views across Union Bay, bird-watching and other wildlife watching

EXPOSURE: Mostly shaded

TRAFFIC: Heavy

TRAIL SURFACE: Dirt, gravel, small amount of boardwalk

HIKING TIME: 1–3 hours

ACCESS: Hikable year-round; no fee for parking or park access

MAPS: USGS Seattle North

FACILITIES: Restrooms and water at the visitor center

■ SNAPSHOT

A few Seattle parks provide a glimpse of the way it used to be by harboring the last stands of the thick forest that once covered the region. The Washington Park Arboretum is a similar sanctuary, instead featuring exotic plant life from around the world. Rather than a trip back in time, the Arboretum allows visitors to take a walk to all corners of the earth via a peaceful system of trails through its carefully manicured gardens and groves.

■ CLOSE-UP

Any hike at the Washington Park Arboretum should begin at the visitor center, where plenty of good information on the park is available through a collection of maps, pamphlets, and handouts. An attached store sells general-interest books on botany, nature, and wildlife, and its helpful staff can assist by answering any questions. The center also occasionally hosts gala events and receptions in the great hall and under the trellis on the patio outside. For anyone seeking a more personal educational experience, the

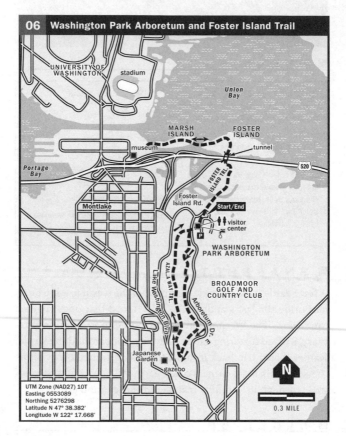

06 Washington Park Arboretum and Foster Island Trail

UTM Zone (NAD27) 10T
Easting 0553089
Northing 5276298
Latitude N 47° 38.382'
Longitude W 122° 17.668'

0.3 MILE

visitor center also offers free guided walks; call (206) 543-8801 for the schedule.

The Arboretum claims to have more than 40,000 plants from 4,600 different species, 139 listed as endangered. Chances are, if something can grow in the climate and soil at Washington Park, a sample will be on display. Many are grouped into named collections, including lindens, camellias, magnolias, Asiatic maples, larches, and numerous others. Several specific exhibits highlight individual classes or geographic areas, such as a rhododendron grove and the New Zealand high country.

Multiple species are identified with signs, listing both common and scientific names. Trees range from the very familiar *Pseudotsuga menziesii,* or Douglas fir, icon of the Pacific Northwest, to the extremely rare *Franklinia alatamaha,* or Franklinia, originally from the state of Georgia and thought to be extinct in the wild since about 1800.

The Arboretum is carefully landscaped with ponds, a gazebo, and plenty of places to stop and reflect. A mix of scents and fragrances fill the air. And although the park is particularly popular during the spring bloom, the wide range of species means that something is at its peak here virtually every month out of the year.

Laid out linearly along a north-south axis, the Arboretum is generally bounded on the east by Arboretum Drive E and on the west by Lake Washington Boulevard E, though some sections spill over the road on either side. In between, a maze of connecting trails wind their way through the heart of the park, allowing visitors to explore the various groves and gardens.

This kind of design does not lend itself well to a single recommended route, however. The best way to see the majority of the Arboretum's displays is to form an elongated loop by traveling south on the trails generally paralleling Arboretum Drive E, then returning on Azalea Way, a broad, grassy path that forms the spine of the park. Side trips to individual areas of particular interest can easily be added to this general framework to suit personal tastes.

Foster Island Trail

A second hiking option—commonly known as the Foster Island Trail, or the Arboretum Waterfront Trail—leads northeast from the visitor-center parking lot. Although passing through what is technically part of the Arboretum, this route explores the marshlands along Lake Washington's western shore and has an entirely different look and feel than the care-fully arranged plant collections in the park's main section.

The trail begins as a dirt-and-gravel road and soon reaches a bridge that crosses a lake inlet to access Foster Island. Pass through the Arboretum's last identified grove of trees and then duck underneath WA 520 through a tunnel, with the traffic humming overhead. Enter a grassy area on the far side, then turn left where the trail narrows into the reeds.

A wooden observation platform is on the right, looking out over the Montlake Ship Canal, Union Bay, and Webster Point at the tip of the Laurelhurst neighborhood across the water. The University of Washington, with its distinctive winged stadium rising unmistakably above the lake, occupies most of the land to the left. At any time of year a steady parade of boats will be pass-ing by. And if the Huskies are in action, an entire armada of loyal supporters unfailingly anchors in the bay.

However, the chief sightseeing attraction here is not the cityscape but the natural environment. Foster Island is an excel-lent bird-watching site, with flocks of ducks and other water-fowl swimming on the lake and congregating among the reeds.

The trail continues on an extensive boardwalk system of wood, metal, and concrete, occasionally crossing out over the water. The lake is very shallow in this area, and it is possible to see the bottom in several places. The boardwalk eventually ends on Marsh Island, where the trail returns to dirt and enters a tangled thicket of mud and stunted trees. Additional opportu-nities abound for observing the island's wildlife, including bea-vers, whose teeth marks are visible on some of the stumps.

At the far end of Marsh Island, the trail crosses back to the mainland on a bridge and reaches its western terminus in the parking lot for the Museum of History and Industry (MOHAI), a total of about 1 mile from the Arboretum's visitor center. From here, it is possible to complete a loop back to the starting point by walking along Lake Washington Boulevard E. This busy road is not well-suited for foot traffic, though; the safer and more scenic option is to return the way you came.

■ MORE FUN

The Washington Park Arboretum also maintains an excellent 3.5-acre Japanese garden, which includes a traditional teahouse. The garden, located at 1075 Lake Washington Boulevard E, is adjacent to the southern end of the Arboretum's main grounds and charges an admission fee. For more information, call (206) 684-4725 or visit the garden's Web site at **www.seattle.gov/parks/parkspaces/japanesegarden.htm.**

■ TO THE TRAILHEAD

From I-5 north of downtown Seattle, go east on WA 520. Take the first exit off WA 520, Montlake Boulevard. Go straight across Montlake Boulevard onto Lake Washington Boulevard E. In about 0.5 miles, turn left onto Foster Island Road, then turn right onto Arboretum Drive E. The parking area at the visitor center is immediately on the left.

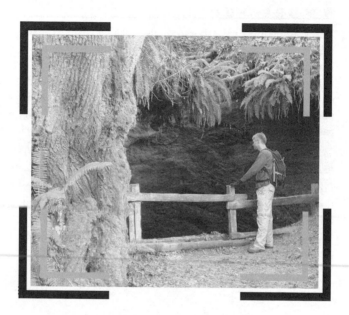

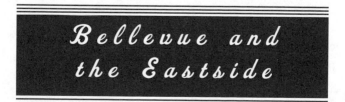

Bellevue and the Eastside

■ OVERVIEW

LENGTH: 2.1 miles (side-trip options)	**HIKING TIME:** 1–2 hours
CONFIGURATION: Figure 8 loop	**ACCESS:** Hikable year-round; no fees for parking or park access
SCENERY: Wetlands, slough, wildlife, blueberry farm, native flora and fauna	**MAPS:** See map at trailhead or pick up pamphlet in Winter House Visitor Center; USGS Bellevue South
EXPOSURE: Mostly open, some shady areas	**FACILITIES:** Restrooms and water at visitor center
TRAFFIC: Popular on sunny days	
TRAIL SURFACE: Mixture of gravel, boardwalk, dirt, and wood chips	

■ SNAPSHOT

This Bellevue Parks and Community Services Department gem offers easy access to a vast array of native plants and wildlife, just minutes from downtown. The vestigial wetlands provide a window into life here prior to modern development. And the interesting site history and working blueberry farm ensure that everyone will find something they'll enjoy.

■ CLOSE-UP

Surrounded by high-rises, rampant suburbs, and two interstate highways, the Mercer Slough Nature Park is a true ecological oasis in the heart of Bellevue. Encompassing more than 320 acres of wetlands and several miles of hiking trails, the location offers a great quick escape for nature-lovers of all kinds.

But don't be fooled; the slough's easy access does not compromise its natural setting. Mercer is the largest urban wetland in King County, and it contains an incredible range of wildlife despite its relatively small size. Mink, otters, beavers, and even coyotes call the park home, along with more than 100 different species of birds, making it one of the most diverse ecosystems in the Puget Sound region.

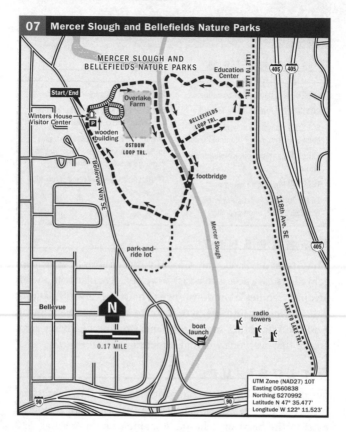

07 Mercer Slough and Bellefields Nature Parks

Before beginning your hike, be sure to stop by the visitor center in the Winters House at the northern end of the parking lot. Listed on the National Register of Historic Places, the Spanish-styled house was built by Frederick and Cecelia Winters in 1929 with funds earned from their on-site nursery. Initially specializing in greenhouse-raised azaleas, daffodils, and irises, the Winters attained success in bulb farming after the spread of an infectious blight led to a quarantine on imports.

The estate was purchased in 1943 by Austrian immigrants

Anna and Frank Riepel; Mrs. Riepel resided in the house until 1983, when it began to fall into disrepair. Five years later, the city of Bellevue purchased the property and restored it to its current condition. In addition to serving as the park's visitor center, the Winters House also is home to the Bellevue Historical Society and serves as a gathering place for meetings, receptions, and banquets.

The hike begins on the eastern side of the parking lot; look for a display board featuring park information and an excellent map. Head north on the gravel path to the start of the Heritage Trail boardwalk. The trail is well marked, but note that on many signs decimal points are missing from the stated distances—0.3 miles looks like 3 miles, for instance.

As you enter the wetlands, the ruins of an old wooden building appear on the right. The structure is falling apart and sinking into the ground, being reclaimed by the mud. Although you are only a stone's throw from Bellevue Way SE, the sounds of birds in the willows begin to overtake the dull roar of traffic.

In less than 100 yards, the Ostbow Loop both starts and ends on the right. Endre Ostbow grew rhododendrons here on land purchased from the Riepels, and the side loop that now bears his name winds through many of these plants still thriving in the bog. Whether you explore this spur or not, at the second intersection follow the main trail to the left, heading north.

The boardwalk passes under a living arch of dogwood branches before bending through a cattail marsh and reaching an abrupt end. A fence separates the neatly planted rows of Overlake Farm blueberry bushes on the right from the wood-chip trail and chaos of natural growth on the left. Like Ostbow's surviving rhododendrons, the blueberry farm connects the developed Bellevue of today with its agricultural roots of the past. Continue along the fence to where a riot of wild blackberry bushes lines the main channel of the slough.

Cross the footbridge over the dark, slow-moving water, watching for kayakers and canoers paddling by. The high-rises of downtown Bellevue are visible just to the north, a reminder of the development that lays siege to this last natural refuge.

Great blue herons often fly overhead or stand in the rushes on the banks here. Despite their striking size and color, these birds can be surprisingly well camouflaged in the reeds. Other bird species you might spot include ruddy ducks, wigeons, buffleheads, hooded mergansers, and mallards. And if you are here during the fall run (September to December), you may catch sight of chinook and coho salmon swimming upstream to spawn.

The boardwalk resumes on the eastern side of the bridge, reaching a T-shaped junction with the Bellefields Loop. Follow the wood-chip-lined trail to the right (east) into shrubs and meadows. Several interpretive displays around the loop provide valuable natural and historical information about the area.

In less than a quarter mile, a group of benches marks a gravel path that enters from the right. Continue on the main trail to the left, past a stand of large western red cedars. These massive trees mark the original eastern shore of Lake Washington, which receded after the construction of the ship canal in 1917. Stay to the left again and cross Trail Creek, bypassing the short hill to the right leading to the Bellefields trailhead on 118th Avenue SE.

On the far side of the stream, the trail splits and you can veer right over a small rise or head left to stay along the lower path. Skunk cabbage lines both trails here; the sight of the plant's yellow flowers helps to offset its thick, unpleasant odor during the spring and summer bloom. Either direction will take you to the next junction, where the trails meet again. From there, continue westward through scrub to reach the edge of the slough, passing viewpoints that offer continued chances to spot wildlife. Returning to the boardwalk, you will complete the Bellefields Loop and arrive back at the footbridge you crossed earlier.

After crossing, stay to the left and continue on the boardwalk. As you navigate the wetlands, be sure to watch for tulips in the thicket. It is amazing that these flowers can capture enough sunlight in the heavy tangle of reeds and brushes to grow. Enjoy the small miracle of these beautiful blooms if you should be lucky enough to see one.

After less than 0.2 miles, a gravel path branches to the right. Leave the boardwalk and follow this path back along the Overlake Farm building and then finally to the Winters House parking lot, where you began.

Note that there are many options for lengthening your hike. A paved biking and running trail circumnavigates the entire park perimeter and joins with the Lake-to-Lake Trail, which connects Lake Sammamish to Lake Washington.

■ TO THE TRAILHEAD

From I-5 just south of downtown Seattle, go east on I-90. Take Exit 9 and follow the ramp as it curves to the north and becomes Bellevue Way SE. Soon you will pass a boat launch, the South Bellevue Park and Ride, and the Overlake Blueberry Farm. Just past the farm, look for the blue Winters House trailhead sign on the right and park in the adjacent lot.

■ OVERVIEW

LENGTH: 2.5 miles (round-trip)	**HIKING TIME:** 2–3 hours
CONFIGURATION: Loop	**ACCESS:** Hikable year-round
SCENERY: Lake Washington shoreline and area; views across the lake; a grotto	**MAPS:** USGS Seattle North
EXPOSURE: Mostly shaded	**FACILITIES:** Restroom and water available near the swimming pool close to the parking area; a great park with large play structures for small children
TRAFFIC: Moderate to heavy	
TRAIL SURFACE: Dirt	

■ SNAPSHOT

This former Catholic seminary sits on a high, forested bluff above the northern end of Lake Washington, providing access to one of the last stretches of undeveloped land on the waterfront via an excellent trail system.

■ CLOSE-UP

Many people primarily know Saint Edward State Park as the host of the annual Washington Brewer's Festival, during which thirsty crowds fill the expansive lawn and eagerly sample the showcased handcrafted beers. The popular event, held each year over the weekend of Father's Day, also features live music, food and craft booths, and even a raucous keg-toss competition.

Yet most of the time Saint Edward is quiet and calm, closer to the contemplative retreat likely envisioned when the seminary was founded by the Sulpician Order in the early 1930s. Named for Edward the Confessor, the second-to-last Anglo-Saxon king of England and founder of Westminster Abbey, the impressive facility was run by the Seattle Archdiocese until it was donated to the state of Washington in 1977 and turned into a park.

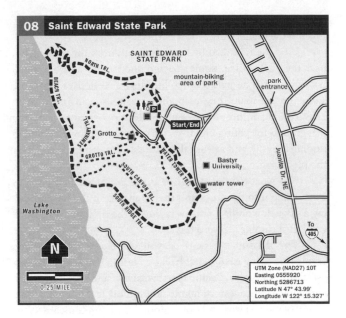

08 Saint Edward State Park

The seminary was built in a Tuscan architectural style, complete with arches and a bell tower, giving the structure a distinctly European flair. The occasional cricket or soccer game on the grass only heightens the atmosphere, extending a general sense of peace that pervades the park. The serenity may reach its apex at the Grotto, an outdoor sanctuary and shrine on the southwest corner of the lawn. This same tranquility is evident throughout Saint Edward's trail network as well.

A counterclockwise loop around the park perimeter is provided by linking the North, Beach, South Ridge, and Water Tower trails, designated almost entirely as "hiking-only." Although Saint Edward is popular with local mountain bikers, who call it Saint Eddy, they tend to stay in the northeast corner of the park near the main entrance and have limited access to Lake Washington and the bluffs, where most of this loop occurs.

Find the trailhead by heading north from the parking lot, past the park office, some storage sheds, and another small parking area. The park's office building also houses a gymnasium (one of many fine recreation facilities available at Saint Edward), in addition to a popular indoor pool and an engaging playground for young children. Park maps can prove helpful in finding the way, and are usually available at a display board near the picnic area.

The North Trail (identified as the Perimeter Trail) begins by ducking into the trees and then bending to the left, following a ridge downhill. A narrow ravine to the right houses a small creek that tumbles toward the lake.

The descent steepens as you get closer to the water, employing some easy switchbacks to lessen the drop. The forest is a mix of typical Pacific Northwest lowland species, including Douglas firs, western hemlocks, and big leaf maples, with a carpet of sword ferns and other ground cover underneath. Gaps in the canopy provide views of the water and the houses of Lake City on the opposite side, a little more than a mile away.

After dropping about 100 feet, the North Trail ends on the lakeshore at a junction with the Beach Trail. Turn left and head south along the bank, where several distinctive red-barked Pacific madrones hang out over the water. Boats frequently pass by, along with float planes from the Kenmore Air Harbor, 2 miles north at the mouth of the Sammamish River.

A thick tangle of plants prohibits easy access to the water until you reach a beachfront clearing with a swimming area along some rocks, where kayakers frequently stop to rest. The wide Seminary Trail enters the clearing from the left; this is the only beach access available to mountain bikers. For hikers seeking a shorter loop, it is possible to return to the main lawn by heading directly up the hill. Just past two lavatories, the Grotto Trail branches off the Seminary Trail to the right, providing another path to the top. At 0.4 miles long, the narrow Grotto Trail is closed to mountain bikes and may be a more rewarding hike than the Seminary Trail.

To resume the Perimeter Loop, continue on the Beach Trail. Bypass the first left to the South Canyon Trail and stay right to join the South Ridge Trail, which quickly climbs above the lake. This trail is surprisingly demanding, running through a series of short ups and downs while ascending a high crest between the South Canyon on the left and a shallower ravine to the right.

Emerge from the woods below a water tower overlooking Bastyr University, a leading center for study of the natural-health sciences. Bastyr now leases the Saint Thomas Seminary, added to the Saint Edward Seminary in 1958 and still owned by the Seattle Archdiocese. The Water Tower Trail starts here, heading immediately left from the wooden gate at the end of the South Ridge Trail and running through the trees along the Bastyr parking lot and access road.

The Plateau Trail enters from the right, open to mountain bikers who may share the broad Water Tower Trail with you the rest of the way. Only about a quarter mile remains until you exit the forest next to the playground and cross the grass to return to your vehicle.

■ TO THE TRAILHEAD

From I-5 just north of downtown Seattle, go east on WA 520. After crossing Lake Washington, go north on I-405 and take Exit 20A, NE 116th Street. Turn left onto 116th Street, which becomes NE Juanita Drive then turns north and changes its name to Juanita Drive NE. Watch for the park entrance on the left (west) side of Juanita Drive NE, which is also the entrance to Bastyr University. After entering the park, stay to the right and park in the main parking lot near the swimming pool building and seminary.

■ OVERVIEW

LENGTH: 1.2 miles (round-trip)	**TRAIL SURFACE:** Dirt, gravel
CONFIGURATION: Loop	**HIKING TIME:** 1–2 hours
SCENERY: Old-growth trees (including a 600-year-old Douglas fir), salmon-spawning creek, historic structures; views of Lake Washington	**ACCESS:** Hikable year-round; no fees for parking or park access
	MAPS: USGS Bellevue North
EXPOSURE: Shaded	**FACILITIES:** Restroom and water at lakefront picnic area
TRAFFIC: Low	

■ SNAPSHOT

At O. O. Denny Park, nothing is as it seems. What looks like a small, lakefront green space in the city of Kirkland is actually a narrow slice of deep forest owned by the city of Seattle. Some of the largest trees in the city stand here, including the broken off trunk of a 600-year-old Douglas fir, reportedly the largest tree in King County until high winds felled it in the early 1990s. An easy trail loops through the narrow creek valley.

■ CLOSE-UP

O. O. Denny Park is largely known for its beach—if it is known at all. With an open picnic area right on Lake Washington, families arrive on hot summer weekends to relax, play, and have barbecues on the grass. A large wooden shelter is often reserved for formal occasions and large gatherings, and a quarter mile of access to the water provides good views of the opposite shore, including the enormous National Oceanic and Atmospheric Administration (NOAA) installation at Sand Point to the south.

Yet even residents of the quiet Juanita neighborhood that surrounds the park seem largely unaware of the astonishing

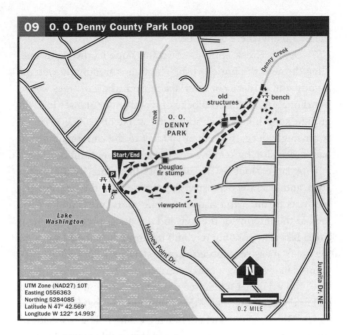

09 O. O. Denny County Park Loop

O. O. DENNY PARK

Denny Creek

Creek

old structures

bench

Douglas fir stump

Start/End

viewpoint

Lake Washington

Holmes Point Dr.

Juanita Dr. NE

N

0.2 MILE

UTM Zone (NAD27) 10T
Easting 0556363
Northing 5284085
Latitude N 47° 42.569'
Longitude W 122° 14.993'

forest that lies along the Denny Creek ravine, across the road from the lake. Even on some of the busiest days, relatively few visitors venture out on the trails and into the woods, missing out on some of the park's most outstanding features.

The trail begins uphill into the trees from the northern side of the parking lot. Within a few hundred yards, a small network of side trails branches to the left to explore a grove of giant western red cedars. These substantial trees are just the beginning of some of the exemplary specimens representing many of the signature species of the Pacific Northwest that can be found in the park. Along with the red cedars, various Douglas firs, grand firs, black cottonwoods, and western hemlocks all stand more than 150 feet tall. Some of the trees rise more than

200 feet, placing them among the largest known samples of their kind anywhere in Seattle.

Denny Creek appears down the slope to the right, bubbling through the underbrush. The trail is frequently wet and muddy and in near-constant shade from the tall trees above, but thoughtfully placed blocks of wood and stone set into the ground keep hikers' feet above the worst of it. The ravine is surprisingly deep, more than 100 feet to the rim, retaining the park's seclusion by keeping nearby development out of sight.

A large Douglas fir lays across the route, spanning the creek and reaching extensively up the bank on the far side. The trail cuts through the trunk near the roots, providing a good look at the interior of the tree and a chance to count its many rings. It is also possible to climb up around the end to inspect the tree's massive exposed root system and speculate on its demise, likely during a heavy storm.

But even that fallen tree cannot prepare you for what you will find just up the trail—the giant trunk of what was once the largest Douglas fir anywhere in King County. The word stump cannot adequately describe what is left of this incredible tree, which still stands more than 60 feet tall and has a base circumference that easily tops 25 feet. Even its bark is impressive, deep and rugged like an inscription from the ages, a testimony to its six centuries of survival and growth. This tree once towered far above the ravine, a condition that unfortunately exposed it to the wild wind that finally brought it down.

Beyond the fallen Douglas fir, an open clearing in a natural amphitheater with a few ruined buildings gives a glimpse into some local history. The park is named for Orion O. Denny, second son of Seattle founders Arthur and Mary Denny, who once owned a country estate on the property. Named *Klahanie,* an adaptation of a Chinook tribal word meaning "the outdoors," the estate was deeded to the city as a public park in Denny's memory by his third wife around the time of World War I. This site was accessible via a gravel road on the far side of the creek, the beginning of the hike's return loop.

This trail continues up the ravine another quarter mile, adding an out-and-back tail to the loop. The route crosses the creek and climbs a few wooden stairs to reach a bench on the southern side of the ravine. Some short switchbacks continue up the slope, eventually ending at the side of a street in the Finn Hill community. A better option is to descend back along the creek to reach an interesting exposed clay wall in the side of the bank, an optimal turnaround point just around the next corner.

Return to the gravel road and cross the creek on a foot-bridge. Local volunteers undertook an extensive habitat-rehabilitation project here in 2002, adding boulder weirs and step pools as part of a man-made fish ladder to help with salmon recovery. Clusters of snake grass and sword ferns run along the creek, along with salmonberry, blackberry, salal, and big leaf maples.

The wide trail climbs toward the top of the ravine, where it ends on a residential street. A view opens out to the south through the trees, encompassing Lake Washington and the eastern end of the WA 520 bridge. After enjoying the view, backtrack 20 yards to find a singletrack trail marked with a post and follow it downhill toward the creek to return to Holmes Point Drive NE, just south of where your vehicle is parked.

■ TO THE TRAILHEAD

From I-5 just north of downtown Seattle, go east on WA 520. After crossing Lake Washington, go north on I-405 and take Exit 20A, NE 116th Street. Turn left onto NE 116th Street, which becomes NE Juanita Drive, turns north, and then changes to Juanita Drive NE. Turn left onto 76th Place NE, which becomes Holmes Point Drive NE. Continue more than 1 mile from Juanita Drive NE, and look for the trailhead parking lot on the right across the road from the O. O. Denny Park lakefront picnic area.

OVERVIEW

LENGTH: 4.6 miles (round-trip)

CONFIGURATION: Loop with side-trip options

SCENERY: Wetlands, plant life, well-maintained hiking trails, and optional interpretive trails

EXPOSURE: Mostly shaded

TRAFFIC: Medium to high

TRAIL SURFACE: Mixture of dirt and gravel

HIKING TIME: 2–3 hours

ACCESS: Hikable year-round; no fees for parking or park access

MAPS: USGS Bellevue North

FACILITIES: Restroom at trailhead; no drinking water available

SPECIAL COMMENTS: Two additional short loops, both natural interpretive trails, are available as hiking options from the parking lot: the Tree Frog Loop Trail runs for 0.3 miles from the eastern side, and the 0.6-mile Trout Loop Trail starts on the western side. It is also possible to string together any number of shorter or longer trips through the preserve on any trail combination of your choosing.

SNAPSHOT

Well-maintained in trails and facilities and yet well-protected from encroaching development, the Redmond Watershed Preserve offers a worthwhile natural experience right on the city's doorstep. A wide network of multiple-use trails explores the reaches of the preserve, providing good hiking opportunities in a surprisingly scenic environment.

CLOSE-UP

The city of Redmond purchased some land from the Weyerhaeuser Corporation in 1926, hoping to use it as a source of water. At the time, the property, in what was then essentially the wilderness, must have seemed a long way outside the city. Although the site never panned out as a suitable watershed (the water was not of sufficient quality), as the city spread eastward the land became valuable for other reasons. What was once a distant piece of backwoods has now become a great outdoor-recreation site right in

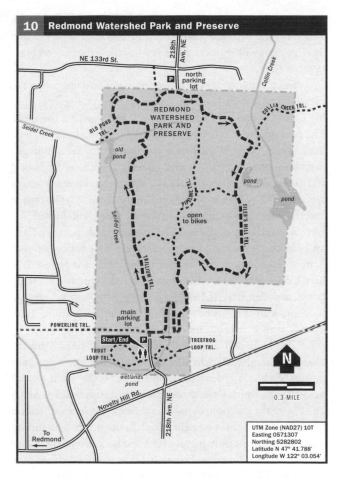

10 Redmond Watershed Park and Preserve

NE 133rd St.
218th Ave. NE
Collin Creek
north parking lot
Seidel Creek
REDMOND WATERSHED PARK AND PRESERVE
COLLIN CREEK TRL.
OLD POND TRL.
old pond
Seidel Creek
PIPELINE TRL.
pond
pond
open to bikes
SILENT HILL TRL.
TRILLIUM TRL.
main parking lot
POWERLINE TRL.
Start/End
TREEFROG LOOP TRL.
TROUT LOOP TRL.
wetlands pond
Novelty Hill Rd.
218th Ave. NE
To Redmond

N

0.3 MILE

UTM Zone (NAD27) 10T
Easting 0571307
Northing 5282802
Latitude N 47° 41.788'
Longitude W 122° 03.054'

Redmond's backyard, and the watershed preserve has, in fact, turned into a forest and wetlands preserve instead.

Nonetheless, the setting is not entirely pristine, as open corridors for overhead power lines and a buried gas pipeline stand as reminders that the area was born to serve the urban population. But even these pieces of civilization are well integrated into the trail system: the two corridors together form the park's backbone and link the preserve to the extended Tolt Pipeline Trail, popular with mountain bikers who follow the path on long-distance rides.

Since 1994, great efforts have been put into upgrading the preserve's recreational facilities, enhancing everything from parking lot bathrooms to bridges, benches, and signs on the trails. The new sign system is now so thorough and the routes so well marked you couldn't get lost if you wanted to. Yet amazingly, despite its proximity to the ever-growing suburbs of Redmond and the good natural experience available, the preserve still seems underused. The city estimates that only about 25,000 people visit the watershed each year—half as many as climb Mount Si.

A grand tour of the park, linking several different trails in an extended 4.6-mile loop, presents the best hiking option. Start at the northern end of the parking lot on the signed Trillium Connector Trail, which heads into the woods on a wide gravel surface. After 0.2 miles, go straight across a four-way junction with the Power Line Trail to join the Trillium Trail, open to hikers and equestrians but not mountain bikers.

The Trillium Trail runs through a forest of second-growth Douglas firs and western hemlocks as it rolls over gentle ups-and-downs. Visible in a depression on the left is the main fork of Seidel Creek, which flows through ferns in the understory. At 0.6 miles from the junction, bypass the Pipeline Connector Trail on the right and continue straight ahead, to the north. The surface underfoot changes from gravel to dirt and back several times, but the trail remains broad and smooth. Cross two footbridges over side forks of Seidel Creek, flowing down from the right.

After the two creek crossings, bend around to the left and reach a junction with the Old Pond Trail, which leads for a quarter mile to an exit onto 209th Avenue. The small pond itself can be seen through the trees on the left, where the three forks of Seidel Creek run together. The marshy land around the pond provides habitat for animals like beavers, great blue herons, and other waterfowl.

Stay on the Trillium Trail by following a tight turn to the right. Then curve through the northwestern corner of the park for about a half mile to reach another junction. Go right on the Pipeline Trail (signed as Collin Creek Trail), which runs parallel to the northern boundary of the preserve. Pass two spurs on the left that head out into the local suburban neighborhood, then bend back toward the center of the park. After another quarter mile you'll reach a junction with the Collin Creek Trail.

Turn left onto the Collin Creek Trail for another 0.3 miles to reach a junction with the hikers-only Siler's Mill Trail on the right. Join the Siler's Mill Trail and pass through a wooden gate designed to keep out horses and mountain bikers. Despite limited access, the trail remains just as wide as on the previous sections.

A pond becomes visible on the left, part of the park's most extensive wetlands ecosystem which is also the source of north-flowing Collin Creek. A second, substantially larger pond lies a quarter mile behind the first on the preserve boundary; it is neither visible nor accessible from here.

The Siler's Mill Trail offers the purest hiking experience in the park, thanks to its restricted access and views of the scenic wetlands. Stay left at a junction just past the first pond to remain on the trail through the rich forest for another 1.1 miles, then pass through another wooden gate and turn left to rejoin the Pipeline Trail, which is open to all users. Follow the pipeline to a major junction with the Power Line Trail and turn right underneath the humming wires. A final 0.7 miles returns you to the Trillium Connector Trail, where a left turn carries you back to the parking lot and your vehicle.

■ TO THE TRAILHEAD

From I-5 in Seattle, take Exit 168B onto WA 520 E. Stay on WA 520 to the end in Redmond, and continue straight onto Avondale Road. After just more than 1 mile, turn right onto Novelty Hill Road. Continue 2.3 miles to the park entrance on the left, across from 218th Avenue NE.

11   Coal Creek Park

■ OVERVIEW

LENGTH: 6 miles (round-trip)	**HIKING TIME:** 2–3 hours
CONFIGURATION: Out-and-back with optional return route	**ACCESS:** Hikable year-round; no fees for parking or park access
SCENERY: Historic mines and structures; waterfalls and a creek	**MAPS:** Green Trails—Cougar Mountain/ Squak Mountain 203S; USGS Bellevue South
EXPOSURE: Shaded	
TRAFFIC: Moderate	**FACILITIES:** No restroom or water at trailhead
TRAIL SURFACE: Mostly dirt; some gravel near trailhead; some boardwalk	

■ SNAPSHOT

It might be hard to believe, but this modest park helped build Seattle. Supplying coal to a rapidly expanding population across the lake, the Newcastle mine that used to operate here fueled the region's explosive growth at the end of the 19th century. Today, the park still serves the city, but as a refuge from the urban sprawl it once spawned, with a trail through a narrow creek ravine leading to two waterfalls and several excellent historical sites.

■ CLOSE-UP

The trail through Coal Creek Park is surely one of the most surprising hikes anywhere around Puget Sound. Featuring several waterfalls, a small canyon, and an environment typical of the Cascade foothills, the park stretches the boundary between the suburbs of Bellevue and the natural areas of the Issaquah Alps, a green finger pointing from the foot of Cougar Mountain through the rows of houses along Lake Washington's eastern shore.

The greater Seattle area is blessed with many excellent urban hikes, each offering a quick escape from the local neighborhood. What makes Coal Creek Park so unusual, though, is

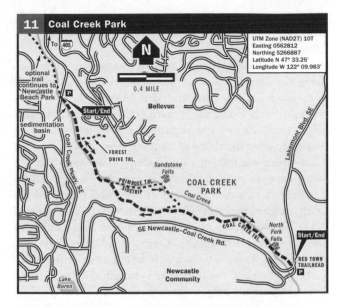

not that it is an undeveloped island in a sea of civilization but that only a century ago it was just the opposite. In the late 1800s, when virgin forest still reached all the way to the shores of Elliot Bay and today's Eastside was mostly untracked wilderness, the park was the site of the Newcastle coal mine—a substantial industrial operation that, if it were still standing, would over- whelm even the busy neighborhoods that currently surround it. As you hike the trail, watch for remaining vestiges of the mining days, clues to the story of Newcastle coal. Yet the most compel- ling story in the park is undoubtedly the extent to which nature has reclaimed the land. Most of the time, it's difficult to imagine that any human development ever took place here at all.

The western trailhead begins at the parking lot, near the chain-link fence protecting the Coal Creek Parkway Sedimen- tation Basin. Built in 1986, the basin is designed to keep the creek channel clear by capturing sediment carried by the water before it can continue downstream; it also provides habitat for fish in several man-made pools and ponds, harboring a variety of trout and salmon species.

The trail narrows to a single-track as the canyon deepens along the northern side of the creek, crossing several side streams running down from the ridge. Although the Coal Creek watershed only drains the western side of Cougar Mountain, which rarely carries a snowpack, the water is usually high enough to cover the sound of the traffic from above.

After a half mile, the Forest Drive Trail enters from the steep slope on the left. Continue past this intersection for another half mile through a mix of brush and trees until you reach a signed junction with the Primrose Trail (numbered N11), allowing you to visit Sandstone Falls and complete a short loop with the main Coal Creek Trail (N1) on the return. Strangely, the trails are not named in an intuitive way and would make more sense if the titles were switched; it is the Primrose Trail which closely follows the creek, not the Coal Creek Trail.

Follow the Primrose Trail along the creek to a site with a few sandstone boulders, a relatively uncommon geologic formation for this area where rocks of volcanic origin are much more common. Reach Sandstone Falls after 0.4 miles, where a side creek slides down over an exposed piece of the underlying sedimentary rock before joining the main channel. Although the 20-foot drop isn't much by high Cascade Mountain standards, it is certainly exceptional by Bellevue standards, especially during periods of peak flow.

The canyon reaches its deepest point just past the falls, and the sides begin to steepen. Watch for some remnants of the old mining operation along the southern side of the creek, including rusty iron cart wheels and a cable partially buried in the dirt.

The trail climbs out of the inner canyon to rejoin the Coal Creek Trail, some 0.8 miles from the previous junction. Turn left and pass below a ridge, notable for the multitude of ferns which seemingly pour down from the top, to the right. The trees soon give way to a small open area at a retired gravel pit, with views of some radio towers and large houses on the western slope of Cougar Mountain. A glance back the way you came might provide a glimpse of the northern end of the Olympic Mountain Range and the prominent Columbia Tower in downtown Seattle, more easily seen in winter when the trees are bare.

Join a dirt road through the clearing, then return to the trail on the far side at a sign for Red Town trailhead. Just beyond the bottom of some boardwalk stairs, look for a concrete slab off to the right, the base of the old locomotive turntable. Surprisingly, the concrete looks as if it was poured yesterday, without significant weathering, yet all other evidence that a busy rail line once ran here has essentially disappeared, swallowed by the woods.

Beyond the turntable, two waterfalls mark the last quarter mile of the trail. Coal Creek pours over a short man-made drop of beams and planks—all that is left of a substantial wooden housing that once enclosed the entire flow—in the creek bed. Mere steps above it, North Fork Falls tumble down a striking slab of red rock on the left, similar in height to Sandstone Falls but much more impressive, with a greater volume of water.

The trail splits nearby, creating a very short loop; be sure to explore both sides. On the north, a rich vein of coal (all that remains of an old mine shaft) is exposed and open for inspection. The opposite side features a fascinating information kiosk on the Newcastle operation from 1867 to 1929. It is almost impossible to imagine that at one time a large hotel stood nearby, locomotives steamed through, and crowds of physical laborers toiled on the very spot you now stand. Several old photographs tell the story, though, revealing the magnitude of the development needed to recover, process, and transport the coal.

Red Town trailhead is just up a short hill, the turnaround point for this hike. Head back the way you came, remembering to stay on the main Coal Creek Trail at the junction for the Primrose Trail to complete the central loop.

Many options are available if you wish to continue farther. Red Town is also one of the most popular places for access to Cougar Mountain, just across the road from the end of the Coal Creek Trail. From the western trailhead where you began, look for a sign to the Lower Coal Creek Trail on the opposite side of Coal Creek Parkway SE. The linear park continues down the canyon as far as Newcastle Beach Park via the Lake Washington Trail, 2.3 miles one way.

■ TO THE TRAILHEAD

From I-5 south of downtown Seattle, go east on I-90. Immediately after crossing Mercer Island and Lake Washington, take the I-405 S exit and stay in the right-hand lane. Then take the first exit—Exit 10, Coal Creek Parkway. At the end of the exit, turn left and go underneath I-405. Continue on this winding road past the Factoria Mall area. At about 1.3 miles from I-405, look for the trailhead parking area on the left (east) side of the road at the bottom of Coal Creek Canyon.

■ OVERVIEW

LENGTH: 3.5 miles (round-trip) plus a 0.6-mile side trip	**ACCESS:** Hikable year-round; no fee for parking or park access
CONFIGURATION: Loop	**MAPS:** Green Trails—Cougar Mountain/Squak Mountain 203S; USGS Bellevue South
SCENERY: Several modest viewpoints and cascading Wilderness Creek	
EXPOSURE: Mostly shaded	**FACILITIES:** Restroom at trailhead; no drinking water available
TRAFFIC: Moderate	**SPECIAL COMMENTS:** This trailhead is prone to frequent car break-ins, so be sure to take your valuables with you, or better yet, leave them at home.
TRAIL SURFACE: Dirt	
HIKING TIME: 2–3 hours	

■ SNAPSHOT

Cougar Mountain receives many visitors, but most are concentrated at the busy Red Town trailhead, far from the mountain's high point at Wilderness Peak. The quiet Wilderness Creek Trail climbs to the park's little-known summit via an appealing valley, passing several viewpoints along the way.

■ CLOSE-UP

Unlike its higher neighbors in the Issaquah Alps, Cougar Mountain has a flat, marshy area as its heart. Where both Squak and Tiger mountains have a clearly discernible central crest, Cougar is more like a plateau, climbing on all sides to reach a broad, even middle. With this unusual topography, the true summit is difficult to discern from a wide range of similar high points among the trees.

Aided both by its drive-up approach and its name, which recalls the mountain's history as a military installation, Anti-Aircraft Peak attracts a lot of attention. However, at 1,483 feet it

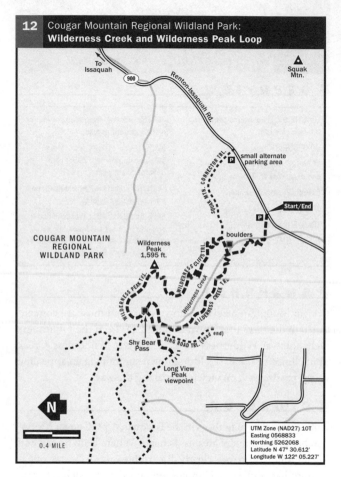

12 Cougar Mountain Regional Wildland Park:
Wilderness Creek and Wilderness Peak Loop

To Issaquah

900

Renton-Issaquah Rd.

Squak Mtn.

small alternate parking area

Start/End

COUGAR MOUNTAIN REGIONAL WILDLAND PARK

SQUAK MTN. CONNECTOR TRL.

boulders

Wilderness Peak 1,595 ft.

WILDERNESS CLIFF TRL.

Wilderness Creek

WILDERNESS CREEK TRL.

WILDERNESS PEAK TRL.

Shy Bear Pass

RING ROAD TRL. (dead end)

Long View Peak viewpoint

N

0.4 MILE

UTM Zone (NAD27) 10T
Easting 0568833
Northing 5262068
Latitude N 47° 30.612'
Longitude W 122° 05.227'

is only the second-highest point on Cougar Mountain, more than 100 feet lower than 1,595-foot Wilderness Peak, about a mile away to the south.

The hike to Wilderness Peak starts from the northwest end of the small parking lot, signed as E6 Wilderness Creek Trail. Note that the letter E indicates that this trail is in the eastern section of the park, a naming convention used throughout Cougar Mountain; other trails can also be preceded by N, W, or S for the remaining compass directions, or C for trails in the center.

Just past the trailhead, a footbridge crosses Wilderness Creek as it splashes down through mossy boulders and logs. The trail then climbs on the southern side of the creek through some short switchbacks, generally with the water flowing within earshot as it heads up the ridge.

Cross back over the creek on a second bridge after about a half mile to reach the first junction, and stay to your left; the right-hand option, signed as Wilderness Creek Trail, serves as the end of the loop on the descent.

Some glacial erratics, not surprisingly known as "The Boulders," soon appear on the right. The big rocks continue intermittently up the slope, inviting speculation on both the massive forces required to deposit them here and the power of erosion that may eventually grind them to dust.

Cross the creek several more times as the trail ascends to a flatter marshy area. Carefully laid wooden planks wind between some more erratics, keeping hikers above the mud and away from both stinging nettles and thorny devil's club, with some particularly nasty specimens reaching more than ten feet high. Past the marsh, the trail starts climbing again through a forest of tall Douglas firs and eventually reaches an important intersection at Shy Bear Pass, elevation approximately 1,350 feet, where several S and E trails converge.

The signed trail to Long View Peak heads left, allowing a 0.6-mile out-and-back side trip to a nearby viewpoint. The overlook is far short of spectacular and typical for Cougar Mountain, with intervening trees and a relatively narrow angle of view; nonetheless, it makes an interesting diversion. To reach the viewpoint, stay on the S4 Long View Peak Trail past a junction with the S5 Ring Road Trail, then turn left onto an unsigned spur where the S3 Deceiver Trail branches to the right. The spur goes up and over a small rise to reach the viewpoint, which looks out over a slice of South Seattle and Puget Sound.

Return to Shy Bear Pass and follow the signed E4 Wilderness Peak Trail on a gentle uphill singletrack to where it crests after about 0.3 miles. Drop down slightly and go past the right turn onto the E5 Wilderness Cliffs Trail. The high point is only another 0.1 mile, where the trail dead-ends at a bench in a circular grove of tall trees. Lacking a view or even a single exposed rock, Wilderness Peak hardly passes for a summit, by most definitions of the word. But the spot beneath the trees is pleasant and peaceful, like a quiet chapel in the woods.

Return to the previous intersection and turn left to start descending the Wilderness Cliffs Trail. The route drops gradually at first, but soon becomes steeper and enters some switchbacks beneath the high Douglas firs. Two viewpoints look out over the May Creek Valley through gaps in the trees—the first just off to the right and the second farther down to the left—although neither provides what could be described as an all-encompassing vista. Wilderness Creek can be heard in the ravine below, too far down to be visible.

The signed Squak Mountain Connector Trail eventually branches off to the left. Stay to the right for another 400 feet to return to the Wilderness Creek Trail at the junction you encountered earlier, closing the loop. From here, continue down the same way you originally came up.

■ TO THE TRAILHEAD

From I-5 south of downtown Seattle, go east on I-90. Take Exit 15 and turn right onto WA 900 West, which begins as 17th Avenue NW and then becomes Renton-Issaquah Road SE. About 3.3 miles from I-90 and just after SE 95th Street is the entrance to a parking lot for the Wilderness Creek trailhead on the right.

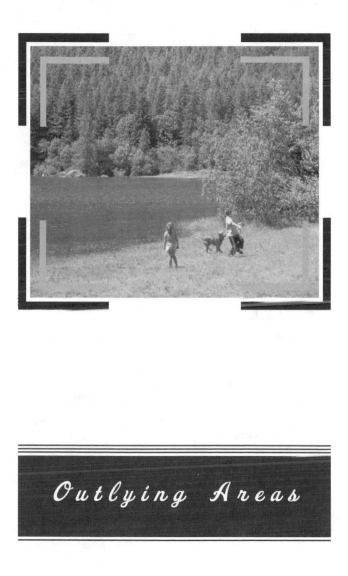

Outlying Areas

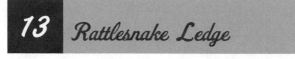

13 Rattlesnake Ledge

■ OVERVIEW

LENGTH: 4 miles	**ACCESS:** Hikable year-round, though Rattlesnake Mountain may be snow-covered in winter; no fees
CONFIGURATION: Out-and-back	
SCENERY: Forest, views, lake	
EXPOSURE: Mostly shaded	**MAPS:** Green Trails—Rattlesnake Mountain Map 205S; USGS North Bend Quad
TRAFFIC: High	
TRAIL SURFACE: Dirt	
HIKING TIME: 2–3 hours	**FACILITIES:** Restrooms near the Rattlesnake Lake parking area

■ SNAPSHOT

Long a popular outing for its proximity to Seattle and commanding views of the Snoqualmie Valley, Rattlesnake Ledge is a well-known hiker's destination. It deserves all the attention it gets, delivering a memorable outdoor experience in a beautiful setting any time of year.

■ CLOSE-UP

In 1911, Seattle closed off the Cedar River Watershed to protect the city's primary source of drinking water, established some 20 years earlier in 1889. For almost a century since, careful stewardship of the pristine waters and surrounding land has left the area largely undisturbed, leaving a semiwilderness right on the doorstep of the now-developed town of North Bend. The elk that occasionally wander through residents' yards are a testament to the still untamed nature of the protected region.

The trails on Rattlesnake Mountain skirt the edge of the Cedar River Watershed and allow the public to get as close to the area as possible without special access. An education center lies along the southern side of Rattlesnake Lake on Cedar Falls Road; it provides information on the natural and human

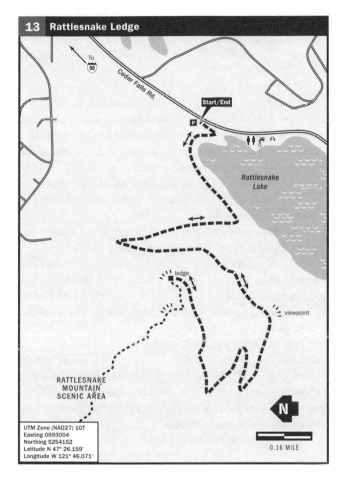

13 **Rattlesnake Ledge**

To 90

Cedar Falls Rd.

Start/End

P

Rattlesnake Lake

ledge

viewpoint

RATTLESNAKE MOUNTAIN SCENIC AREA

UTM Zone (NAD27) 10T
Easting 0593004
Northing 5254152
Latitude N 47° 26.159'
Longitude W 121° 46.071'

N

0.16 MILE

history of the region along with an overview of many of the issues surrounding water storage and use and can easily be reached via a lakeshore trail that originates at the parking lot and is open to foot traffic and bicycles.

The ample parking area is well developed and offers special lots for boat trailers and handicapped access. Many visitors come only to spend a day at the edge of the lake for a barbecue and swim, or to paddle a canoe on the water. No overnight camping is allowed, though, and the gates are closed and locked each night at 9:30.

The crowds of today are no anomaly; this area has seen regular human use for close to 10,000 years, starting when the first Native Americans arrived. Establishing routes around what was then a tall-grass prairie, they came from nearby settlements in search of berries, herbs, animals, and fish. Although the source of the Rattlesnake name remains unknown, it possibly dates back to these early inhabitants. The lake remains an important site for modern Native Americans and is stocked with rainbow trout.

The hikers-only trail starts as a gravel road from the southwest side of the parking lot; it's marked with a large sign. Note that although the trail is never hard to find or follow, the signage is often inconsistent and inaccurate. The information board and map by the lakeshore fail to show any of the Rattle-snake Mountain trails beyond the ledge, and distances tend to be underestimated.

Find the true trailhead a few minutes along the gravel road to the right. From this point, it is 2 miles one-way to Rat-tlesnake Ledge and a climb of 1,175 feet. Several signs here also give conflicting information, so look for the newest ones that show the correct distance. Similar signs along the way correctly mark each half mile to the ledge.

The trail starts on a gradual climb through a forest of moss-covered trees and ferns, with the occasional boulder or stump along the way. The Douglas firs are particularly impres-sive here, some reaching more than 100 feet tall with diameters of less than four feet. Their lack of low-level branches yields a pleasing display of strong vertical lines. The well-worn trail continues to gain altitude as it leads through a series of broad switchbacks up the slope.

Immediately before the 1-mile mark, a viewpoint opens out to the left, revealing views deep into the watershed protected area. Rattlesnake Lake and the education center appear to the southwest, with Mount Lindsay beyond.

A short downhill section follows, the only relief from the relentless climb which soon begins again. No-trespassing signs hang on some of the trees on the side of the trail to mark the watershed boundary. A few more long switchbacks lead to a junction that's signed and marked with a map.

The fork to the right leads to Rattlesnake Ledge, just a few steps away at an elevation of 2,080 feet. Considered the eastern terminus of the Issaquah Alps, the rocky ledge has a commanding view of almost 270 degrees, including the entire lower Snoqualmie Valley. Rattlesnake Lake and distant Chester Morse Lake sparkle below Cedar Butte and Mount Washington.

This is a great place to sun yourself on a rock and enjoy the view; arrive in the morning to take advantage of the southeastern-facing aspect. However, be careful of your footing, especially when hiking with children, as a deep chasm runs through the center of the ledge and cliffs drop off on all sides.

After visiting the ledge, return the way you came.

■ TO THE TRAILHEAD

From I-5 just south of downtown Seattle, go east on I-90. Take Exit 32, 436th Avenue SE, and turn right (south). The road becomes Cedar Falls Road and winds for more than 2.5 miles to a large sign for Rattlesnake Lake; turn right off Cedar Falls Road here. Immediately make another right into a parking lot signed for Rattlesnake Ledge Trail Parking. If this lot is full, there are many more spaces in the southern lot next to the lake.

14 Little Si Trail

■ OVERVIEW

LENGTH: 4 miles	**TRAIL SURFACE:** Dirt with rocks, roots
CONFIGURATION: Out-and-back	**HIKING TIME:** 2–3 hours
SCENERY: An easier alternative to Mount Si with similar views of North Bend and the Snoqualmie River Valley	**ACCESS:** Hikable year-round; no parking fees
EXPOSURE: Mostly shaded	**MAPS:** Green Trails—Mount Si NRCA Map 206S; North Bend USGS Quad
TRAFFIC: High on weekends	**FACILITIES:** Restrooms at the trailhead

■ SNAPSHOT

Long overshadowed literally and figuratively by its big brother next door, Little Si is finally getting the attention it deserves. Little Si is a worthwhile destination on its own and makes a great alternate when its hulking neighbor is too busy, too socked in, or too demanding.

■ CLOSE-UP

From a distance, it can be hard to even identify Little Si as a separate peak from Mount Si proper. So complete is Mount Si's dominance over the area that the insignificant-seeming bump in front seems hardly worth noticing.

A closer view reveals that this is all a trick of perspective. The minor notch that separates the peaks is actually a deep cleft, and the tree-clad summit ridge of Little Si actually hides impressive cliff faces far more sought by climbers than any on the exposed rock of the bigger peak next door. For hikers, the manageable distance married with a moderate elevation gain presents a solid challenge, although well short of extreme.

Little Si's attractiveness for rock climbers plays a big role in the tight trailhead parking area, especially when the rock is dry. The good news is that this means even when the lot is full

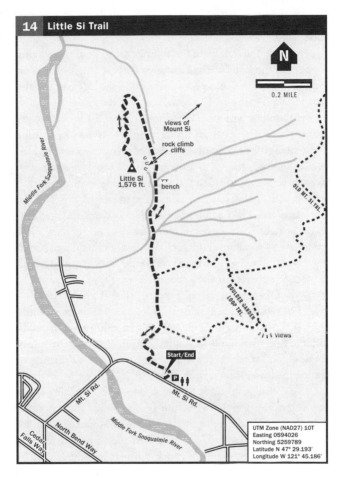

14   Little Si Trail

views of
Mount Si

rock climb
cliffs

Little Si
1,576 ft.

bench

OLD Mt. SI TRL.

Middle Fork Snoqualmie River

BOULDER GARDEN
LOOP TRL.

Views

Start/End

P

Mt. Si Rd.

Mt. Si Rd.

North Bend Way

Cedar
Falls Way

Middle Fork Snoqualmie River

0.2 MILE

N

UTM Zone (NAD27) 10T
Easting 0594026
Northing 5259789
Latitude N 47° 29.193'
Longitude W 121° 45.186'

the trail itself will probably be less crowded than you might think. The bad news is that more often than not there will be a considerable volume of cars to contend with.

The trailhead has space for more than 40 vehicles, but on some days you may need to head for the overflow parking in a gravel lot next to the bridge over the middle fork of the Snoqualmie River.

Start up the trail from the southeast corner of the parking lot, behind the toilets. Right away you face a tough incline on rocks and dirt. A glance back over your shoulder across the broad Snoqualmie River Valley reveals the long ridge of Rattlesnake Mountain, with pockets of radio towers marking its many peaks. The sun here can be brutal, thanks to thin growth and a south-facing slope. Luckily, a series of switchbacks soon lead into some shady trees and ferns where the trail levels out. The forest here is typical of the western Cascade foothills, with a primary mix of Douglas firs, alders, and maples.

After about half a mile, the Boulder Garden Loop branches off to the right. This junction can be tricky to identify since it is unsigned and sometimes obscured by logs or other debris, but it is well worth finding. The loop trail winds past some giant rocks in a section of beautiful, mossy forest. Along the way, stay straight where the Old Mount Si Trail heads uphill to the right.

The return of the Boulder Garden Loop to the main Little Si Trail is clearly signed, making this second junction much easier to find than the first. A good option would be to explore the Boulder Garden on the way down, avoiding the difficulty of finding the lower intersection altogether.

To continue up Little Si, descend to a creek crossing as the trail enters the gap between the peaks. Views start to open through the trees onto the southwest face of Mount Si, with the summit of Little Si now left. An information board marks the first of many access points for rock climbers into the Mount Si Natural Resource Conservation Area, available for day-use only.

The canyon between the two Si's is defined on its western side by a long wall of rock below the Little Si summit ridge, where climbers test their skills. Several vantage points offer the opportunity to stop and watch them tackle the challenging routes and listen to their voices carry through the trees.

A memorial bench dedicated to Doug Hansen provides a

place to sit along the way. Hansen was a popular Seattle-area mountaineer who honed his skills in the high Cascades and ended up being killed along with 11 others on Mount Everest in May 1996. The events were tragically immortalized in Jon Krakauer's *Into Thin Air.*

Past the bench the trail starts to climb again, now heavily shaded below the rock wall. Even on a hot summer day the temperatures are surprisingly cool here, where the sun never really penetrates. After reaching an old rockslide on the left, the trail enters a beautiful fern valley, a mix of dappled greens, sunlight, and shadow. Look for some of the ferns hanging off boulders along the wall and spreading like a carpet over the forest floor.

At the northern end of the valley, the path swings hard to the left and steeply uphill. Unfortunately, the bulk of the climbing on this trail occurs in the last third of its distance as the route exits the valley and mounts the summit ridge, doubling back in the direction you've already come. Prepare for a near-scramble through a few short sections.

When you finally reach the summit, you will feel like you have come a lot farther than the actual distance. Various ledges surround the high point; poke around for a while to find the one that suits you best. Don't miss the rocks slightly down the far side, which have some of the best views over North Bend and where mountain goats can occasionally be spotted. There are also several viewpoints just before the top looking over at Mount Si, clearly showing its much larger size. Stay back from the edge, and be careful not to knock anything off that could hit the rock climbers directly below. The return route is the way you came in.

■ TO THE TRAILHEAD

From I-5 south of downtown Seattle, go east on I-90. Take Exit 32 and turn left (north) onto 436th Avenue SE. Turn left onto SE North Bend Way and then turn right onto SE Mount Si Road. Just after crossing the river and rounding a bend to the right, look for the trailhead parking area on the left signed for Little Si.

OVERVIEW

LENGTH: 2.5 miles (round-trip) or longer	**TRAIL SURFACE:** Dirt; gravel on Iron Horse Trail
CONFIGURATION: Out-and-back	**HIKING TIME:** 2–3 hours
SCENERY: Waterfalls, old-growth trees, river viewpoints, riverside access	**ACCESS:** Hikable year-round; parking area hours 6:30 a.m.–dusk
EXPOSURE: Shaded	**MAPS:** Green Trails—Mount Si NRCA Map 206S; USGS Chester Morse Lake
TRAFFIC: Moderate to heavy; go mid-week for less traffic	**FACILITIES:** Restroom at trailhead

SNAPSHOT

Located well below 2,000 feet and just off I-90, Twin Falls makes a great year-round destination, especially when winter snows close many of the hikes farther up toward Snoqualmie Pass. This hike follows the rocky south fork of the Snoqualmie River and climbs to two significant waterfalls before connecting to a larger network of trails exploring Olallie State Park.

CLOSE-UP

Mention Seattle and the first thing people think of is rain. The city is almost universally identified as one of the wettest places anywhere in the United States, despite the persistent efforts of the Washington State Tourism Department to dispel this image; travelers are invited to the Emerald City with the lure of only 36 inches of annual rainfall, less than such so-called dry places as New York (47 inches) or Atlanta (48 inches). And don't tell the sunbathers and scantily clad club-hoppers at famous South Beach, but the joke is on them: Miami receives 59 inches a year, some 50 percent more than Seattle.

The difference is that, where other cities receive most of their rain in concentrated downpours, Seattle usually sees mist and drizzle that lasts for days but doesn't add up to much, leav-

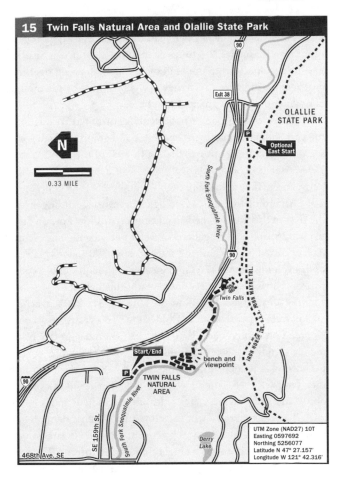

15 Twin Falls Natural Area and Olallie State Park

N

0.33 MILE

Exit 38

OLALLIE
STATE PARK

Optional
East Start

South Fork Snoqualmie River

90

Twin Falls

IRON HORSE TRL. a.k.a. JOHN WAYNE TRL.

Start/End

bench and
viewpoint

TWIN FALLS
NATURAL
AREA

90

SE 159th St.

South Fork Snoqualmie River

468th Ave. SE

Derry
Lake

UTM Zone (NAD27) 10T
Easting 0597692
Northing 5256077
Latitude N 47° 27.157'
Longitude W 121° 42.316'

ing endlessly cloudy skies for nine months out of the year—
almost 300 days, on average—but limited total rainfall
accumulations. Just 30 miles east, however, the region lives up
to its reputation.

The lower western slope of the Cascades is probably the
second wettest place in the state, trailing only the western side

of the Olympic Peninsula. Although no match for the Hoh Rain Forest at 140 inches per year, the Twin Falls region gets more than 90 inches, 2.5 times as much as downtown Seattle. The heavy clouds from the Gulf of Alaska that sweep over the city, keeping it gray but relatively dry, get trapped by the mountains and dump their precipitation here.

However, the rain is not evenly distributed throughout the year, falling primarily in the winter and going through wide seasonal variations. In turn, the south fork of the Snoqualmie River rises and wanes as well, showing a remarkable range between the flow at low and high water.

According to the U.S. Geologic Survey gauge at Edgewick, the river in this area reached an all-time record-low flow on September 28, 2001—172 gallons of water per second. The record high occurred on November 24, 1990, at 80,790 gallons per second, a volume almost 470 times greater. Although this is a comparison between extreme values, yearly fluctuations also show amazing disparities. The flow on January 31, 2003, reached 44,359 gallons per second, 141 times the 314 gallons per second recorded on September 6 later that year. Even day-to-day readings can wildly oscillate; November 18, 2002, saw 1,571 gallons per second, a number that jumped to 14,288 the next day, and then fell back over the next week to less than 1,500. All of this occurs in a small drainage area of less than 65 square miles.

The character of Twin Falls is naturally dependent on the flow of the river. At high-water periods, typically in late winter and spring, expect to see a single thundering torrent. The low water of late summer and fall presents a much more peaceful display, as the falls split into several separate braids. This hike may well warrant several trips at different times of the year to appreciate the full range of experiences available.

The trail starts out winding along the bank of the river. When the flow is suitable, watch for whitewater kayakers who come here to hone their skills by "playboating" sometimes only a stone's throw from the parking lot. About a quarter mile along, some big boulders shelter several potential swimming holes.

Licorice and sword ferns testify to the volume of rain that falls here, but the thick canopy created by the tall Douglas firs can keep the worst of it from reaching the ground, making this a better option than it would seem for hiking during the frequently questionable weather.

Climb through a few long switchbacks to arrive at a high point with a handrail and a bench. The bench faces out toward the lower falls, offering a view that's best in winter when the leaves have fallen from the nearby trees to provide a clear line of sight. Continue down the far side of the ridge and stay left at a junction to reach a giant old-growth fir that dwarfs the other trees around it. This is the first of several such trees, true forest outliers in terms of their monumental size, scattered along the trail.

Another short climb brings you to a set of wooden steps on the right, leading down to an overlook. A fenced platform provides a great straight-on view of the lower falls, where the river is channeled through a narrow gap in the basalt and then spills out over a rocky face, tumbling into a pool below.

Continue for another few hundred yards up the main trail to reach a boardwalk and bridge over the river. This bridge crosses just above the lower falls and provides a good view of the multiple stages of the upper falls, a series of plunge pools dropping through a narrow chasm. A curtain of mist billowing around the corner hints at the top level of the falls, which unfortunately is very difficult to observe from anywhere on the trail.

The bridge makes a good end point, for a total of 2.5 miles round-trip when you reach the parking lot. For a longer hike, continue on the far side of the river for about a half mile to reach a junction with the gravel Iron Horse Trail. Although this section of the trail is pleasant and well maintained, it rises far enough above the river gorge to be exposed to the sound of the traffic on I-90. It's so close, in fact, that occasional glimpses of asphalt and cars appear through the trees.

Adventurous hikers can continue eastward along the Iron Horse for several miles into the heart of Olallie State Park. This extended hike would make an excellent one-way journey with a shuttle; the eastern trailhead is at Exit 38, to the right off I-90.

■ TO THE TRAILHEAD

From I-5 south of downtown Seattle, go east on I-90. Take Exit 34 and turn right (south) onto 468th Avenue SE. In a short distance, turn left onto SE 159th Street. The parking lot for Twin Falls Natural Area is at the end of this road.

For the alternate Olallie State Park trailhead, take Exit 38 and turn right. Go a short distance and take the first right into the signed Twin Falls and Iron Horse Trail parking area.

OVERVIEW

LENGTH: 4 miles plus optional northern-island trails	**HIKING TIME:** 2–4 hours
CONFIGURATION: Loop (figure-eight)	**ACCESS:** Hikable year-round during daylight hours; no fees for parking or park access
SCENERY: Wildlife-watching and bird-watching, wetlands, interpretive boardwalk trails, river and mountain views	**MAPS:** USGS Everett
EXPOSURE: Mostly exposed	**FACILITIES:** Restroom at nearby Langus Riverfront Park; no drinking water available
TRAFFIC: Medium	
TRAIL SURFACE: Mixture of dirt, gravel, pavement, and boardwalk	

SNAPSHOT

Spencer Island sits at the center of the biologically flourishing Snohomish River Estuary, home to countless animals and plants, including more than 350 known species of birds. A series of trails explores the rich life of the wetlands—great for naturalists, bird-watchers, and hikers.

CLOSE-UP

Just north of downtown Everett, freshwater from the mouth of the Snohomish River mingles with the salt water of Possession Sound, creating a highly dynamic environment and forming a critical habitat for hundreds of species. However, these same dynamic forces are frequently not so kind to the land itself. Rising and sinking saltwater tides coupled with seasonal flooding cause the ground to endlessly shift and erode, only to be built up somewhere else. Sitting at the center of the estuary, Spencer Island often gets the brunt of the relentless waters, and in many ways it continues to exist thanks only to an extensive series of dikes and levees designed to keep the river and the ocean at bay.

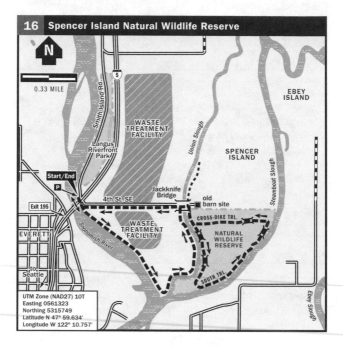

16   Spencer Island Natural Wildlife Reserve

The system is certainly not fail-safe, though, and the largely wood-chip dikes are in constant need of repair. The fragility of the system was graphically displayed in 2003, when catastrophic damage from several large breaches and a fire smoldering within one of the dikes caused the closure of several key trails and significantly altered the landscape. Although two key bridges were finally rebuilt in 2008, recovery and construction work—both to repair the considerable damage and also for ongoing maintenance to prevent further problems—still continue and should be expected for the foreseeable future.

Just as the island sits at the center of the swirling waters of the estuary, so too does it lie in the middle of a mix of government jurisdictions, creating a strange juxtaposition of conflicting uses. The southern half is administered as a Natural Wildlife Reserve by Snohomish County Parks and Recreation, while the northern half, run by the Washington Department of Fish and Wildlife, is open for hunting in season. Yet even with this apparently paradoxical division, the island remains a great place to explore the fascinating Snohomish Estuary.

From the parking lot, there are two different ways to reach the island. The most direct route is on Fourth Street SE heading straight to the Jackknife Bridge, a little more than a half mile away to the east. However, a more interesting route to the bridge leads along the river to the south on the Langus Waterfront Trail and then back up the shoreline of the Union Slough, about 1.5 miles altogether.

The Langus Waterfront Trail promises little in the way of a natural experience at the start, as it is fully paved and almost directly under I-5. The first half mile is only marginally better, with significant industrial development on the far shore and the path bordering the Everett wastewater facility on the left. The exposed treatment pools can occasionally be glimpsed through the trees, and unfortunately the odor tends to waft over the trail unless merciful winds blow it back the other way.

However, things start to improve a little farther along, where tangled blackberry bushes and some benches appear on either side. By the time you reach Union Slough after 0.8 miles, the setting becomes much more pleasant. Follow the slough northward through grasses, reeds, and trees, looking out over the southern end of Spencer Island just across the water to the right.

Jackknife Bridge spans Union Slough where the trail rejoins Fourth Street SE from the parking lot. Cross the bridge to reach the island at a well-signed junction on the far side. The ruins of a barn once sat straight ahead among a sea of cattails, but almost nothing remains of the structure, which was once the heart of the now-closed cattle-ranching operation that spawned the original set of dikes to hold back the water. A boardwalk near the old barn site leads to an interpretive sign.

It was once possible to complete a 3.5-mile grand loop all the way around the perimeter of the island, but the damage to the dikes in 2003 unfortunately eliminated that popular route.

However, it is still possible to complete a smaller loop around the island's bottom half, linking the South Trail and the Cross-Dike Trail. These trails are in the natural reserve and away from bicyclists, dogs, boats, and hunters, so they are sure to provide the most attractive option for the majority of hikers.

Start south on the dirt trail, a right turn as you step off the bridge. Another short interpretive boardwalk leads to an over-look on the left, with excellent views over the reeds; helpful information about the marsh ecosystem is provided by easily noticeable displays. On a clear day, a chain of prominent peaks is visible in the Cascades, including Whitehorse Mountain, Three Fingers, and Mount Pilchuck, with Mount Baker rising far to the north. If the wind is calm, look for reflections of the snow-clad peaks in the still waters below.

Just past the boardwalk, the Cross-Dike Trail leads off to the left on a raised berm through the center of the island. For now, continue along Union Slough on the South Trail. Soon you will reach a bridge (likely seen earlier from the Langus Waterfront Trail on the opposite bank) that may host bird-watching photographers. The bridge provides a flat and stable tripod platform, necessary for the use of giant zoom lenses.

Bend around to the left at the bottom end of the island, now following Steamboat Slough on the uneven levee surface. Some dilapidated houseboats and barges float on the opposite bank and other occasional watercraft go by. A collection of snags stands along the trail here, formed when the trees were inundated by water over the breached levees and subsequently died. The trees' loss is the bird-watchers' gain; all manner of avian species like to perch in the bare treetops, especially hawks, eagles, and other raptors that use the high vantages to look for food. Partway up the trunks, man-made bat boxes provide shel-ter for winged hunters of an altogether different kind.

A newly constructed bridge connects the South Trail to the end of the Cross-Dike Trail. Hike over the bridge and then turn left onto the dike itself to explore the heart of the island on the raised embankment, crossing another new bridge along the way. With no vegetation other than the low reeds, panoramic views of the area are available on all sides, providing some of the best opportunities for wildlife observation anywhere at Spencer. Ducks and a host of other waterfowl are impossible to miss any time of year. Also, deer, beavers, and even seals and otters can occasionally be spotted.

After completing the Cross-Dike Trail, a short walk north returns you to the Jackknife Bridge. From here, it is possible to head straight back to the parking area by following Fourth Street SE and completing the loop, or you may retrace your steps around the longer Langus Waterfront Trail to the left. You also can head along the near side of Union Slough for a short distance to explore the northern portion of Spencer Island.

■ TO THE TRAILHEAD

From I-5 in Everett, take the Marine View Drive exit (Exit 195) and turn left onto East Marine View Drive. Continue north on Marine View Drive (which soon merges with Walnut Street) for about 1.5 miles, then turn left up the curved entrance ramp to WA 529 over the Snohomish River Bridge toward Marysville. Take the first right, then immediately turn right again following signs to Langus Riverfront Park. Turn left at the stop sign at Ross Avenue and continue past the marinas to another intersection and veer right onto Smith Island Road. At the southern end of Langus Riverfront Park is a parking lot and trailhead under I-5.

Meadowdale County Park and Beach

■ OVERVIEW

LENGTH: 2.5 miles (round-trip)	**TRAIL SURFACE:** Mixture of dirt and gravel
CONFIGURATION: Out-and-back	
SCENERY: Lunds Creek and Gulch, Meadowdale Beach, playfields, and a variety of trees with identification plaques	**HIKING TIME:** 1–2 hours
	ACCESS: Hikable year-round; no fees for parking or park access
	MAPS: USGS Edmonds East
EXPOSURE: Shaded along the trail, exposed at the beach	**FACILITIES:** Restroom at trailhead; no drinking water available
TRAFFIC: High	

■ SNAPSHOT

Meadowdale is a valuable rarity among the many good Puget Sound beachfront parks, thanks to restricted road access to the shore. This makes it a great choice for hikers who will enjoy the descent on an easy trail along Lunds Creek, which runs through a beautiful forest on the way to the beach.

■ CLOSE-UP

Not surprisingly for a waterfront parcel of land in the heavily developed Edmonds region, Meadowdale Park passed through many private hands before being acquired by the Snohomish County Parks and Recreation Department in 1968. Of the private owners, the most significant was surely the Meadowdale Country Club, which built and maintained a clubhouse, swimming pool, and other facilities on site, although most of the evidence of the club is long gone. The memory of John Lund, an early homesteader in the late 1800s, is more obvious today— the hike runs through Lunds Gulch, carved out over the ages by the waters of Lunds Creek.

The trail, which starts on the opposite side of the parking lot from a good-sized madrone tree, curves around a broad

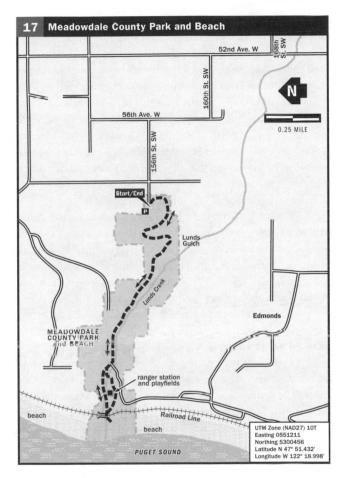

17   Meadowdale County Park and Beach

bend through the field to the east. Start down the wide surface, circling through the grass, and then enter the forest. The gradual descent and smooth trail make this hike a good option for families with small children, who will find the route interesting but not too difficult.

Some wooden stairs and a split-rail fence mark the beginning of a steeper descent into the narrow valley of Lunds Gulch. The fern-covered walls rise 200 feet to the rim, and Lunds Creek soon appears in a gully to the left as the trail runs beneath a mix of maples, Douglas firs, cottonwoods, and alders. Despite its very limited length, the creek carries a number of species of fish, including some salmon that make the run upstream from the ocean to spawn. The mix of freshwater and salt water at the creek's mouth acts as a tiny estuary, where the young smolts go through the substantial physical changes that allow them to make the transition from life in the freshwater of their birth to the salt water of their adult lives, the unique adaptation of anadromous fish.

Moss-covered big leaf maples now seem to be the dominant tree species in the forest, but a series of enormous western hemlock stumps near the half-mile mark give some idea of what the original ecosystem here might have been like. Look for the old springboard notches in the wood, used to support the working platforms the loggers used to fell the ancient giants. A few low-to-the-ground interpretive signs help identify some of the major plant species and point out their distinguishing characteristics, such as the heart-shaped leaves of the black cottonwood.

As you near the beach, high alders lean out over the trail from either side, creating an effect similar to a towering arbor trellis. The setting is magical when the sunlight filters through the majestic living archway to the ground below. The trail emerges from the trees and then crosses the creek on a bridge next to a park ranger station on the left. A road connects the ranger's facility to surface streets on the southern side of the gulch, but access is currently restricted, keeping the crowds away. Only disabled individuals who would otherwise be unable to descend the longer trail from the top are permitted to use this approach. Pass through a grassy clearing with a picnic shelter and a volleyball pit and then duck into a short concrete tunnel under railroad tracks to finally reach the beach.

Lunds Creek empties into Possession Sound through the sand, depositing the sediment and runoff it has collected along its course. At low tide, a tiny barrier island serves as a breakwater just offshore. And numerous small tide pools are exposed, ripe for examination. Pieces of sun-bleached driftwood are scattered around the gravelly beach, cast up by the whims of the tide.

Much like the more-popular beaches at Golden Gardens and Carkeek Parks to the south, Meadowdale is a great place to watch the sun set over the Olympic Mountains. Just to the northwest, Possession Point marks the extreme southeastern end of Whidbey Island, and the northern tip of the Kitsap Peninsula sits straight out to the west.

Spend any length of time along the water, and there is a good chance that a freight train will come thundering up the tracks. The sight and sound of the locomotives hauling a mile-or-more-long chain of cars certainly does not enhance the wilderness aspect of the hike, but the spectacle is thrilling nonetheless.

The beach serves as a frequent haul-out site for harbor seals that come up on shore from the water to help regulate their body temperatures, interact with other individuals, and rest or sleep. Young pups that have not yet learned to fear people are particularly vulnerable while on land and should not be disturbed, especially if they are nursing. Seals may potentially be found here at almost any time of year.

After exploring the beach, retrace your steps up Lunds Creek to the trailhead. You will need to climb back up the 400 feet lost on the descent to complete the round-trip journey of approximately 2.5 miles.

■ TO THE TRAILHEAD

From I-5 north of Seattle, take Exit 183, 164th Street SW, and turn left (west). After 164th Street SW curves south onto 44th Avenue W, turn right onto 168th Street SW, which immediately crosses over WA 99. Turn right onto 52nd Avenue W, then turn left onto 160th Street SW. Turn right onto 56th Avenue W, then turn left onto 156th Street SW and proceed straight into the Meadowdale Park parking lot.

18 *Point Defiance Park*

■ OVERVIEW

LENGTH: 3.6 miles (round-trip)	beaches and viewpoints
CONFIGURATION: Loop	**TRAIL SURFACE:** Dirt
SCENERY: Urban trail through old-growth forest, historic Fort Nisqually, rhododendron garden, sandy beaches; views across Puget Sound	**HIKING TIME:** 2–3 hours
	ACCESS: Hikable year-round; no fees for parking or park access
EXPOSURE: Mostly shaded	**MAPS:** USGS Gig Harbor
TRAFFIC: Medium on trails, high at	**FACILITIES:** Restrooms and water throughout the park

■ SNAPSHOT

Considered Tacoma's backyard playground by many local residents, Point Defiance offers just about everything any hiker could want: historical sites, great views, deep forest, and sandy beaches, all accessible via an extensive network of trails. A loop around the Outside Perimeter Trail will confirm the park as one of the finest urban green spaces anywhere, a natural treasure not far from Tacoma's downtown core.

■ CLOSE-UP

Point Defiance got its name when an early explorer noted that the prominent peninsula held such an advantageous position that a fort on the site could stand against any conceivable invading force. The federal government agreed with that assessment, and in 1866 the land was appropriated for defense of the young Washington Territory, which had been carved out of the larger Oregon Territory in 1853. The land remained a military installation for many decades as the city of Tacoma grew just to the south.

By the time Washington had been admitted to the Union as the 42nd State in 1889, however, the possibility of war in

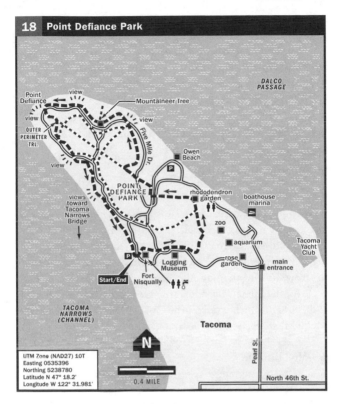

18 Point Defiance Park

DALCO PASSAGE

Point Defiance

view

Mountaineer Tree

view

OUTER PERIMETER TRL.

view

view

Five Mile Dr.

Owen Beach

P

POINT DEFIANCE PARK

rhododendron garden

boathouse marina

views toward Tacoma Narrows Bridge

zoo

aquarium

Tacoma Yacht Club

P

Logging Museum

rose garden

main entrance

Start/End Fort Nisqually

TACOMA NARROWS (CHANNEL)

Tacoma

N

Pearl St.

UTM Zone (NAD27) 10T
Easting 0535396
Northing 5238780
Latitude N 47° 18.2'
Longitude W 122° 31.981'

0.4 MILE

North 46th St.

Puget Sound against the British or any other significant foreign power was growing increasingly remote, and the need for the continuing fortification of Point Defiance became far less apparent. In a victory for local citizens, the land was turned over to the city in 1905 and reborn as a public park, whose first century of existence Tacoma celebrated in 2005.

Ironically, Point Defiance now attracts rather than repels invaders, the multitudes who come every day to take advantage of the park's 700 acres of attractions. On a typical summer weekend Point Defiance is particularly popular, which can make parking difficult, especially near the main entrance. However, there is usually ample space available in the interior along Five Mile Drive. The lot at Fort Nisqually is a good starting point for a hike because it typically has room even on the busiest days, although it is possible to begin from anywhere on the loop.

The Outer Perimeter Trail runs on the top of the bluff all the way around the peninsula and can be hiked in either direction, although it is typically traveled counterclockwise, mirroring the general flow of traffic on Five Mile Drive, which follows a similar route.

Look for the start of the trail on the eastern side of the parking lot away from the water, in the trees beyond the bathrooms and picnic area. The trail is generally well marked with short wooden posts, particularly useful at many points where the hike crosses the road, although some of the posts are concealed by underbrush. Look for a painted square, and possibly an arrow showing the way. Alternate symbols will also appear, a circle for the Spine Trail and a triangle for the Inside Perimeter Trail, both of which intersect the Outer Perimeter Trail and frequently share sections of the route.

After leaving Fort Nisqually, the trail runs gradually downhill through a shady forest of big trees—majestic examples of many signature species of the Pacific Northwest—including hemlocks, cedars, and firs, with a carpet of ferns underneath. After a half mile, pass through the rhododendron garden, where a multitude of azaleas and rhododendrons generously donated by private citizens are on display. The garden is particularly stunning in spring when the plants are in bloom.

A quarter mile past the rhododendrons, cross the Owen Beach access road, which heads down the hill to the right. The beach is a long stretch of sand with a waterfront promenade and a grassy picnic area, invariably busy on sunny days.

Continue along the eastern side of the peninsula to a view of Vashon Island, just across the stretch of water known as

Dalco Passage. Some of the finest old-growth forest in the park stands along this section of the trail, culminating in the impossible-to-miss Mountaineer Tree, a massive, 400-year-old Douglas fir rising more than 200 feet into the sky. Just before the giant tree, watch for a side trail marked with a green square heading down the bluff. It leads to a secluded beach below, great for exploring when the tide is out.

Pass several more viewpoints around the northern tip of the peninsula and then bend back toward the south. Amazingly, although Point Defiance is less than a mile across for most of its width, there is a noticeable difference between the environments on either side. The eastern bluff (which actually faces northeast) is wetter than the western bluff, which has considerable southern exposure. The trail surface underfoot reflects the difference, changing from frequently muddy to more sandy and dry as the trail heads around the point. The plant growth changes as well, with the western side featuring thinner forest and a higher density of the distinctive red-barked madrones.

The Outer Perimeter Trail follows the edge of the bluff on the western side more closely than it does on the eastern, providing repeated views over Puget Sound and the Narrows. The Tacoma Narrows Bridge is visible to the south, gracefully spanning the waters between Tacoma and Gig Harbor. A second bridge parallel to the first was completed in summer of 2007 and is now in full service. It is a safe bet that neither the new concrete structure nor the older steel one will suffer the fate of the infamous original Tacoma Narrows Bridge, affectionately known as Galloping Gertie, which collapsed from a spectacular torsional failure brought on by high winds in November 1940. Engineering students around the world now study the structure as a lesson in how not to design a suspension bridge.

Finish the loop by hiking along the bluff and reach Fort Nisqually where you began.

■ MORE FUN

Point Defiance Park has a host of additional popular attractions, including the Tacoma Zoo and Aquarium, the reconstructed Fort Nisqually site, the Camp Six Logging Museum, an award-winning rose garden, and a boathouse and marina on Commencement Bay. For more information, visit the Point Defiance Park Web site at **www.metroparkstacoma.org/page.php?id=24.**

■ TO THE TRAILHEAD

From I-5 in Tacoma, take Exit 132, WA 16, toward the Tacoma Narrows Bridge. Exit WA 16 before the Tacoma Narrows Bridge at the Sixth Avenue Exit and turn left onto Sixth Avenue at the bottom of the ramp. Cross underneath WA 16 and then immediately turn right onto Pearl Street (WA 163). Continue on Pearl Street all the way to the main entrance of Point Defiance Park. Drive straight into the park and follow the counter-clockwise loop roads to Fort Nisqually and park in the large lot there.

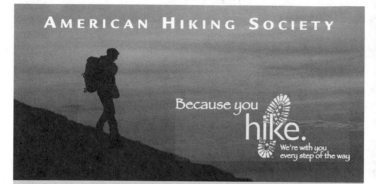
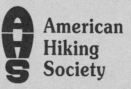